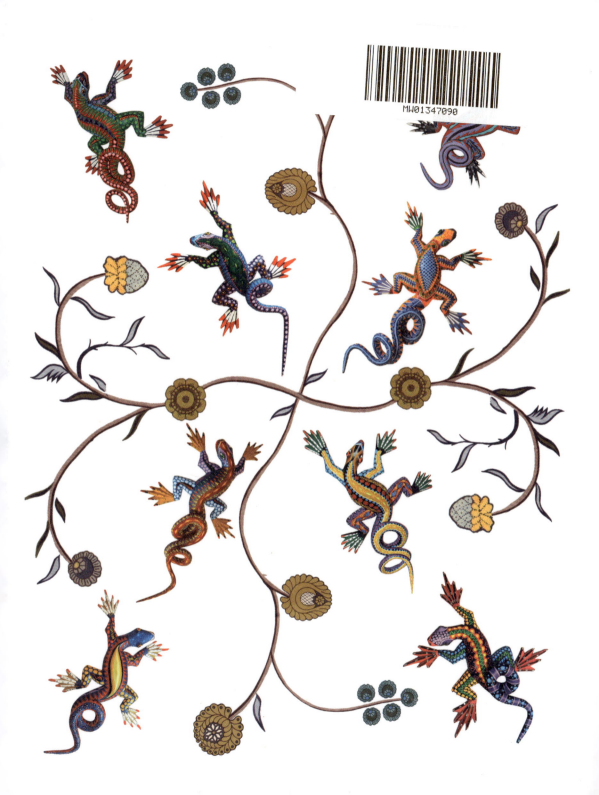

# PLANTS
## IN THE
## MAYAN CULTURE

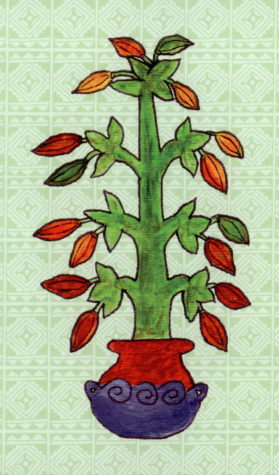

**Traditional Remedies, Food & Art**

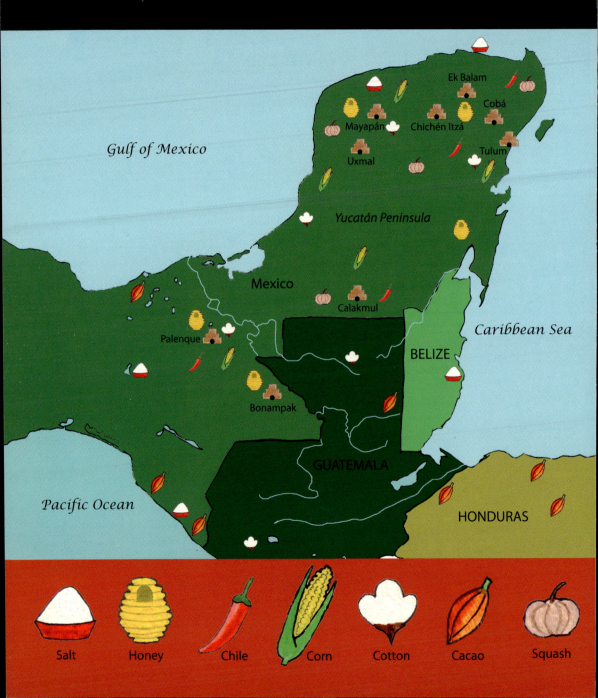

# PLANTS
## IN THE
## MAYAN CULTURE

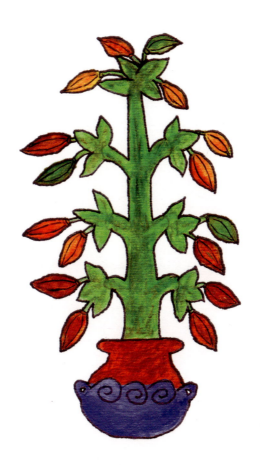

**Traditional Remedies, Food & Art**

First published in 2011
Playa del Carmen, Mexico

ISBN: 978-0-615-39528-9

Copyright © Svetlana V. Aleksandroff 2010

All rights reserved. No part of this publication may be reproduced in any material form (including photocopying or storing it in any medium by electronic means and whether or not transiently or incidentally to some other use of this publication.) without the written permission of the copyright owner.

Note from the publisher
This book contains general information and is not meant to advise or replace any treatment of your preferred health care practitioners. This book provides references that may be used for further research and consultations with trained professionals in order to be applied to gain health benefits.

Art Director: Svetlana V. Aleksandroff
Text: Svetlana V. Aleksandroff
Illustrations: Anna Aleksandroff, pages 64, 100, 260
Vasily Aleksandroff, pages 1, 2, 18, 26
Graphic Design: Vasily Aleksandroff
Photography: Vasily Aleksandroff, Svetlana Aleksandroff

Printed by IMAGO
1st Edition 2011
Playa del Carmen, Mexico

# ACKNOWLEDGEMENTS

This book is a tribute to nature and an expression of our appreciation of it.

During the 5 years that it took us to complete Plants in the Mayan Culture we greatly appreciated the support from the family and some very special friends. We are particularly grateful to Valentina Aleksandrova for her love and support, and Rebeca Torres Castilla for sharing her wisdom and knowledge. We have much gratitude to so many people who were patient while we took photographs in their homes, stores, gardens and workshops and to a special group of people who contributed their faith, enthusiasm and support during the final stages of this project: ............................eneste, Miguel Quintana, Annie Arroyo, Eddy Van Belle, Jeanette Rigter, Genoveva Garcia, Mathieu Brees, Javier Aranda Pedrero, Walailuck Kongsawat, Rosa Maria Vargas and Vasily Izumchensky.

We thank our sponsors, who share our vision of sustainability and care for the planet and who have contributed all the resources for the printing of the first edition of this book: Hacienda Tres Rios, Grupo Xcaret, Fundación Maroma, ........................................, Banyan Tree Spa Mayakoba, Eco-Museum of Chocolate on Plantation Tikul, Choco-Story museum in Bruges - Belgium and Snackbag Co. of Playa del Carmen.

The publishing of this book was possible due to the creativity, talent and dedicated work of Vasily Aleksandroff, our photographer and graphic designer.
We also thank the readers for the interest in our book.

Playa del Carmen
Quintana Roo, Mexico
August 10, 2010

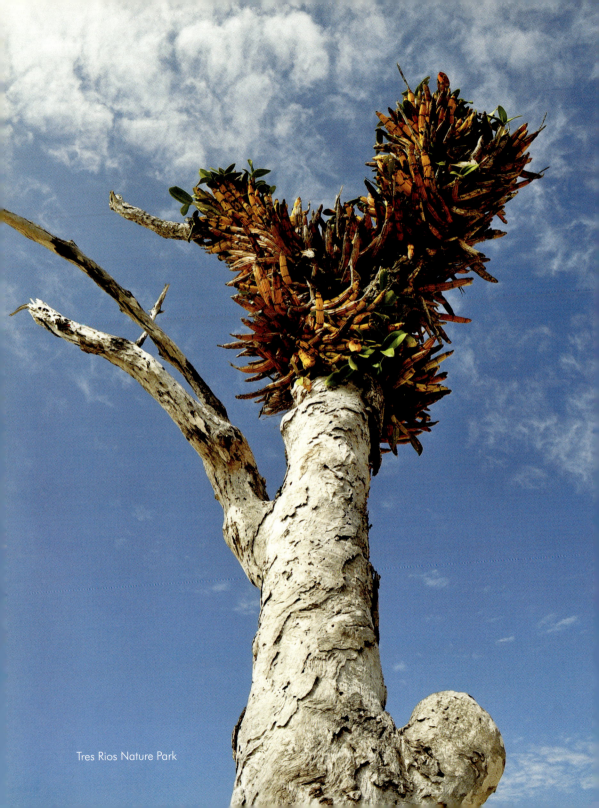
Tres Rios Nature Park

# INTRODUCTION

While I was growing up my grandmother had a beautiful garden on a small piece of land with flowers, apple and cherry trees, vegetables, strawberries and herbs. We were taking care of it as a summer activity and we enjoyed it as a privilege and as a very rewarding experience. I believe that plants are extremely intelligent and sensitive beings capable of bringing to us a range of benefits and experiences that have inspired artists, poets and scientists for many thousands of years.

I was preparing to publish a book about plants for the most of my adult life while studying, doing research, collecting material and books and making and using plant based remedies from my childhood and from the countries in which I lived or traveled.
Learning about the cuisines of different cultures supported my interest in the connection between food and health, introduction of healthy options into the diet in a pleasurable way, combining healthy and enjoyable experiences for the double benefit.

In the year 2004 I was interested in a course called "Herbolaria Maya" taught in Tulum by a friend and herbalist Maria Galindo. After taking this course and learning more about the local plants I decided to start working on a book that would show the great place that plants hold in human society, integrating the medicinal and other uses of plants in one edition with the Mayan culture as an example.

In this book I provide general botanical information about the plant, its traditional use in herbal medicine and in art and culture. Most plants are common to the Yucatan peninsula and the coast of Quintana Roo. The flora in this region is very abundant and unique: the sealine area has mangroves and plants that tolerate salty soil, it continues into an old grown jungle with natural wells, cenotes, and beautiful lagoons, where roots of the trees reach deep between the rocks to get to the underground water, and tree trunks are covered with vines, bromeliads or orchids and there is wild growing pitahaya, passionfruit and prickly pears. Having a combination of native plants, like chaya, achiote or henequen, and many introduced ones, like mango, tamarind, aloe vera resulted in the creation of the unique cuisine, on one hand, and diversified herbal medicine, on the other.

Food has always been one of the important pleasures in my life, and cooking –
a passion, well appreciated by my family and friends. Living in many different countries, absorbing the rich flavors of Mexican cuisine for over 10 years and exploring native Mayan ingredients in healthy variations suitable for the modern palate – resulted in over 50 recipes, that I included in this book, all fast, and easy to make. Preparing food and eating it, both pleasurable activities, can be used to a great benefit for the physical body, if done properly and with love and enjoyment. Learning about food and nutrition is most important for any human being who wants to lead a happy and healthy life.
Make plants your friends and love your food!

Svetlana Aleksandroff
Playa del Carmen, Mexico
November 30, 2009

# Contents

## Chapter 1: Trees of the Forest

| | |
|---|---|
| Anona<br>Cherimoya | 13 |
| Banyan Tree<br>Chac, The Rain God | 17 |
| Cenotes, Tres Rios Nature Park | 19 |
| Bitter Orange | 23 |
| Cacao | 25 |
| Caimito<br>Hog Plum | 29 |
| Coconut Tree | 31 |
| Elephant Ear Tree<br>Breadnut | 35 |
| Fig Tree<br>Serret | 37 |
| Geiger Tree | 39 |
| Guava | 41 |
| Huaya<br>Custard Apple<br>Bay Cedar | 43 |
| Mamey<br>Grosella | 45 |
| Mangrove, Red | 47 |
| Native Hardwood | 51 |
| Sapodilla Tree<br>Mayan Ball Game | 53 |
| Saw Palmetto | 57 |
| Soursop | 63 |
| Tamarind | 65 |
| Tropical Almond<br>Breadfruit | 67 |
| Trumpet Tree | 69 |

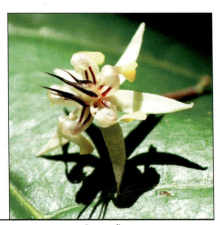

Cacao flower

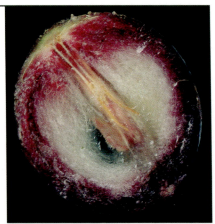

Caimito fruit

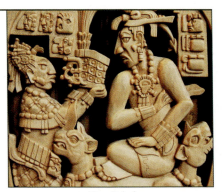

King Pakal

## Chapter 2: Fruit of the Jungle

| | |
|---|---|
| Avocado | 75 |
| Banana<br>Tamales | 77 |
| Dragon Fruit | 83 |
| Lime | 87 |
| Mango | 89 |
| Nopal | 93 |
| Papaya | 97 |
| Pomegranate | 99 |

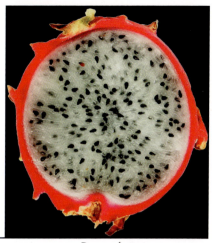

Dragon fruit

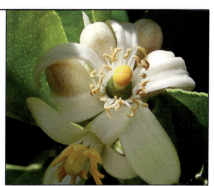

Lime flower

## Chapter 3: Sacred Plants

| | |
|---|---|
| Copal Tree<br>Alebrijes | 103 |
| Corn<br>Nixtamal | 109 |
| Kapok Tree<br>Tree of Life | 121 |
| Squash<br>Arts & Crafts, Musical Instruments | 125 |
| Tabacco<br>Cigars | 135 |
| The Sacred Calendar | 137 |
| Verbena<br>Ixchel | 139 |

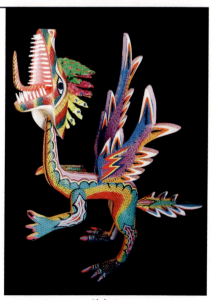

Alebrije

# Chapter 4: Roadside Plants

| | |
|---|---|
| Annato<br>Guaje | 145 |
| Arnica<br>Scorpion's Tail | 147 |
| Bee, Mayan Melipona | 149 |
| Black Poisonwood<br>Castor Oil Plant | 155 |
| Boat Lily<br>Miracle Leaf | 157 |
| Bougainvillea<br>Golondrina | 159 |
| Bromeliads<br>Pineapple | 161 |
| Bull Hoof<br>Pogodo Tree<br>Sanango | 165 |
| Century Plant | 167 |
| Cotton | 179 |
| Firebush<br>Natural Clay<br>Mayan Clay | 191 |
| Flamboyant<br>Basket & Mat Making | 197 |
| Gumbolimbo Tree<br>Ayoyote | 201 |
| Hibiscus<br>Ponche | 203 |
| Orchid<br>Vanilla<br>Coffee | 205 |
| Passion Fruit<br>Passion Flower | 215 |
| Periwinkle<br>Bienvenida | 217 |
| Sea Grapes<br>Railroad Vine | 219 |
| Spanish Needle<br>Wild Balsam Apple | 221 |
| Thornapple | 223 |
| Water Lilly | 229 |

Annato seed pod

Henequen artifacts

Wild passion fruit flower

# Chapter 5: Garden Plants

| | |
|---|---|
| Aloe Vera | 223 |
| Basil<br>Salt | 237 |
| Black Bean<br>Lima Beans | 239 |
| Chaya | 241 |
| Chiles of the Yucatan | 245 |
| Garlic<br>Swiss Chard | 249 |
| Lemon Grass<br>Ginger | 251 |
| Mexican Pepper Leaf<br>Cilantro | 253 |
| Mexican Sage<br>Incense Burner | 255 |
| Mint<br>Sugarcane | 259 |
| Onion<br>Leeks, Scallions, Shallots<br>Polkan | 263 |
| Oregano<br>Turmeric | 267 |
| Root Vegetables<br>Jicama<br>Yuca<br>Yam<br>Ñame | 269 |
| Rosemary<br>Thyme | 273 |
| Rue<br>Obsidian Tools | 275 |
| Tepín Chile<br>Chayote | 277 |
| Tomato<br>Tomatillo | 279 |
| Wormseed<br>Papadzul | 281 |

Aloe vera flower

Polkanes

Purple yam

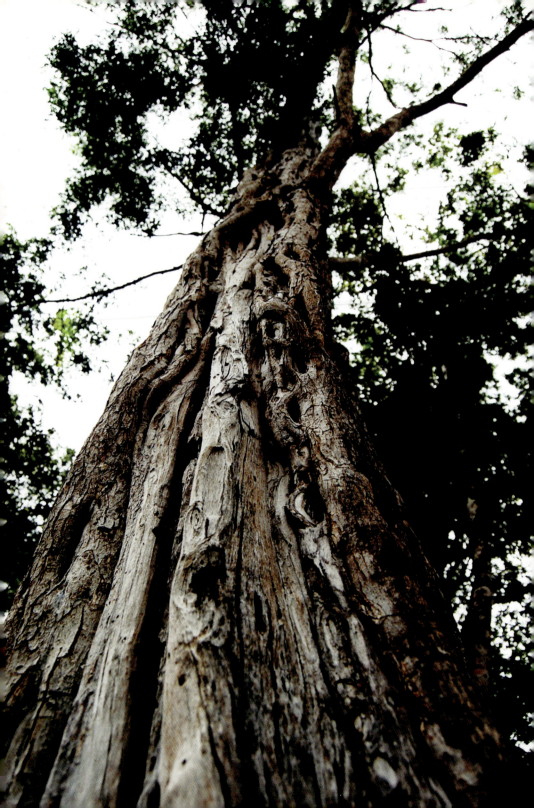

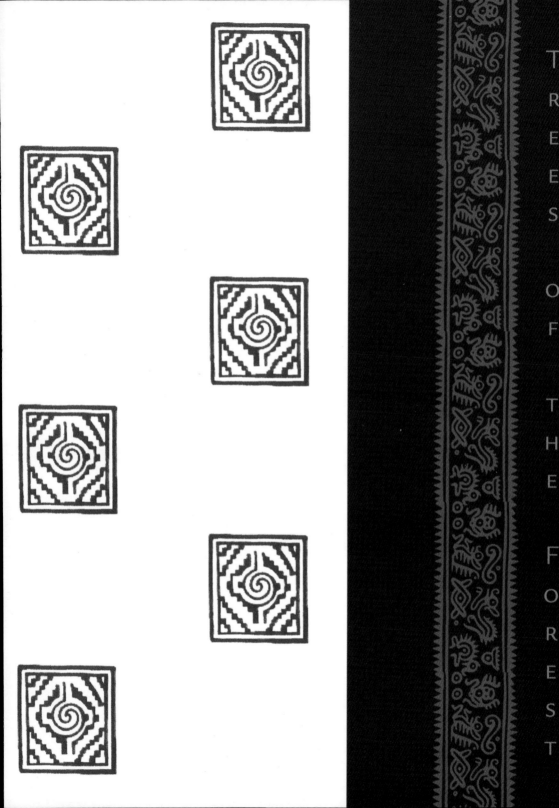

TREES OF THE FOREST

# Anona

### Spanish Name: Anona
### Scientific Name: Annona reticulata L.

Anona is highly nutritious and is an excellent food for children or people who are weak or recuperating from a disease, especially recommended for people with anemia or malnutrition because it is digested very easily.

Juice from fruit may be used as a remedy for common colds and to bring down fevers.

Warmed fruit pulp is a remedy for rheumatisms and may be applied directly to the affected area.

Anona is a tree that originated in tropical America. It survives dry conditions easily and in some parts is as common as pineapple or banana. Along with its close relative, cherimoya, it is appreciated for its juicy, creamy and delicious white pulp with an exquisite aroma similar to cinnamon. Its flavor becomes alleviated if the fruit is cooled off before eating. There are several varieties; the most common in Mexico are white and red.

"When pathogens are strong, the physician should use medicinal herbs to attack and dispel. When the body is deficient, the physician should use dietetics to supplement and fortify."
Huang Di, The Yellow Emperor

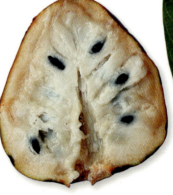

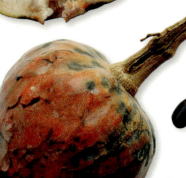

Fruit and seeds

# trees of the forest

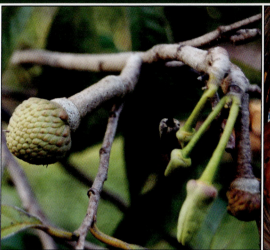
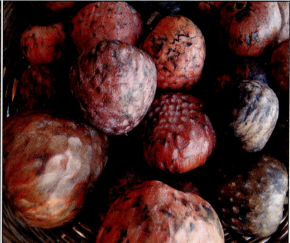
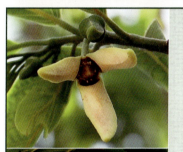
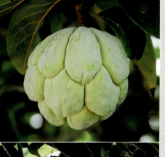

## Chirimoya
### Annona cherimola

Chirimoya is a variety of white anona and is very abundant in Mexico. It is believed to be native to the highland valleys of the Andes. It is a small tree, reaching up to 7 m in height with branches starting close to the ground.

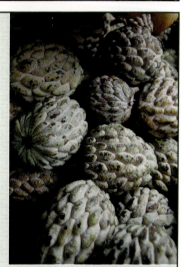

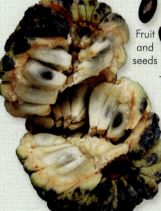

Fruit and seeds

The pulp of the fruit is white and very tender with high sugar, vitamin C and protein content.

The seeds are poisonous and when crushed open and mixed with water may be used as a plant insecticide.

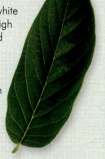

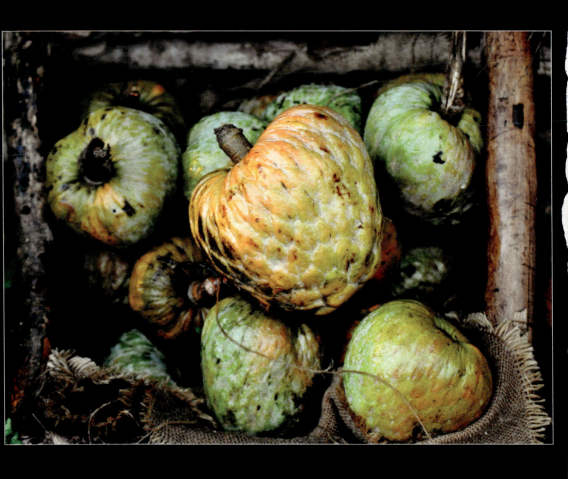

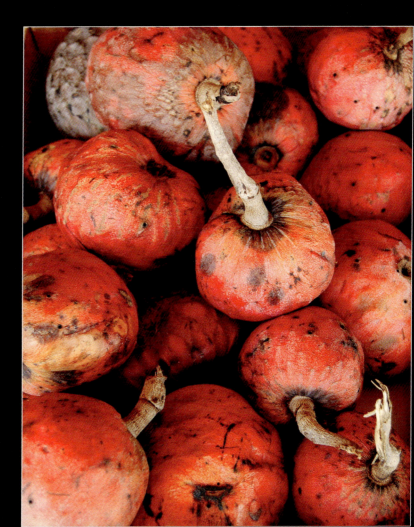

# Banyan Tree

## Spanish Name: Amate
### Scientific Name: Ficus benghalensis

All parts of the tree have been used in traditional medicine since times immemorial.

The white latex is toxic and has been used to treat warts, lumbago and rheumatism.

It was a popular belief that young tender roots of the banyan tree dried and taken on certain days of the menstrual cycle were a good remedy for female infertility.

Young leaf buds were used for dysentery and chronic diarrhea.

A warm poultice made of fresh leaves was applied for minor skin abscesses and sores.

Bark infusion was used as a remedy for diabetes.

The banyan tree is believed to have originated in India. One tree can spread around by growing roots off its branches that turn into new tree trunks. Banyan trees can live for several hundreds of years, reaching the height of 30-35 m. In India the banyan tree is considered to be sacred. The Central American variety, Ficus Pertusa, is native to the American continent and is very common in the Yucatan Peninsula. The tree very often grows near cenotes, or natural wells, with its roots penetrating the bedrock to reach subterranean rivers.

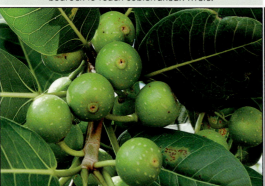
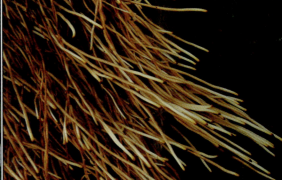

# trees of the forest

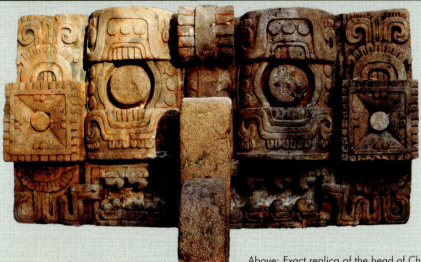

## Chac
### The Rain God

Above: Exact replica of the head of *Chac* carved in order to be placed at the site of the organically grown cacao Plantation Tikul by Belcolade, home to the Eco-Museo del Cacao.

*Chac*, sometimes also referred to as *Chaac* or *Chak*, is an important Mayan deity honored and invoked regularly by farmers to this day. *Chac* is associated with water and rain which results in fertility and good crops and is often represented as an old man with long fangs and an axe, with which thunder is produced. Some drawings show *Chac* fishing in cenotes from a canoe or with a face resembling that of a frog.

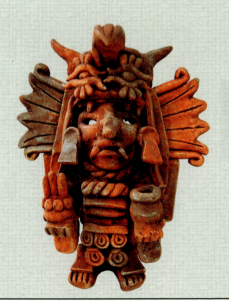

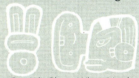

Sac Xib Chac: White-North

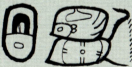

Ek Xib Chac: Black-West

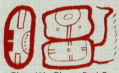

Chac Xib Chac: Red-East

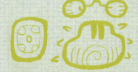

Kan Xib Chac: Yellow-South

*Chac* deities were also very important keepers of the four cardinal directions.

# Tres Ríos Nature Park

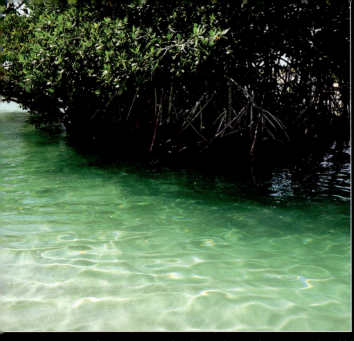

Cenotes, or natural wells, were considered a source of life and were frequently used as ceremonial sites during the ancient Mayan civilization.

The Tres Ríos Nature Park, covering an area of 150 acres, is forever preserved from human impact and construction. The nature park is one of its kind: three rivers run through it forming 10 cenotes with clear and pristine waters and flowing into the sea. It is also unique in having three distinct ecosystems: jungle, mangrove forest and coastal dunes.

Four types of mangroves: red, yellow, white or buttonwood and black along with many other plants are included into the extensive reforestation program. Protected from development, mangroves form a thick coastal barrier, which shelters the hotel from tropical storms and prevents soil erosion.

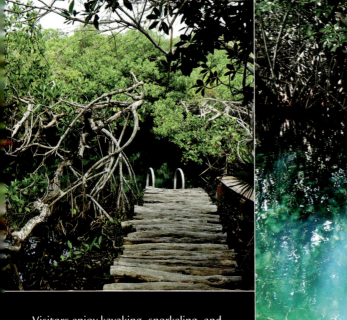

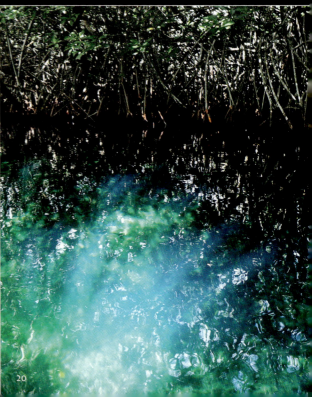

Visitors enjoy kayaking, snorkeling, and excellent wildlife photography opportunities.

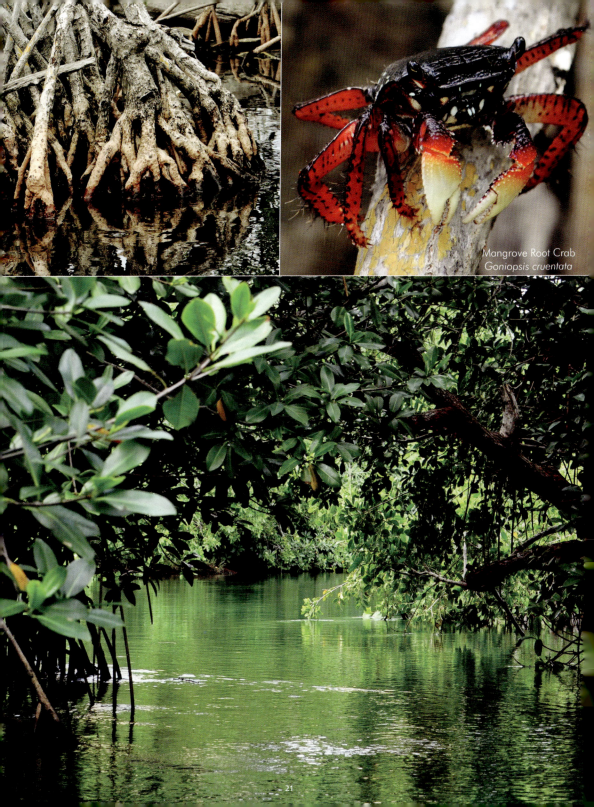

Mangrove Root Crab
*Goniopsis cruentata*

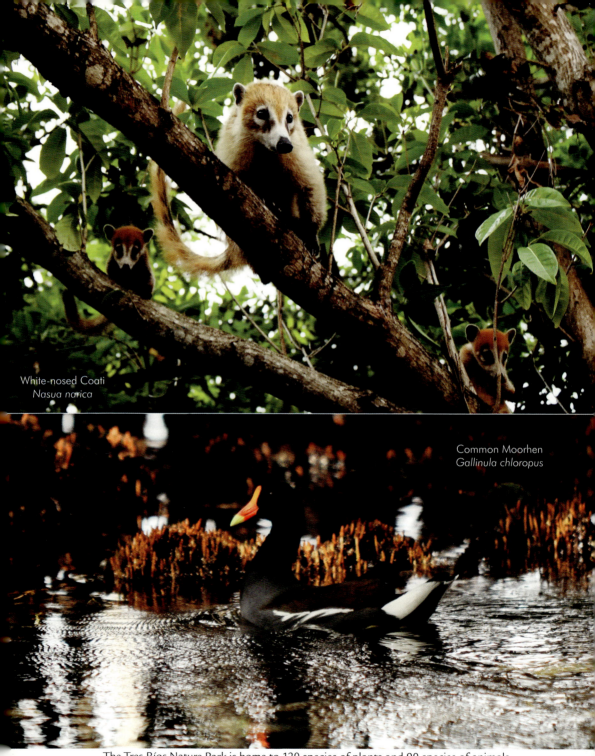

White-nosed Coati
*Nasua narica*

Common Moorhen
*Gallinula chloropus*

The Tres Ríos Nature Park is home to 120 species of plants and 90 species of animals, many of which are in danger of extinction.

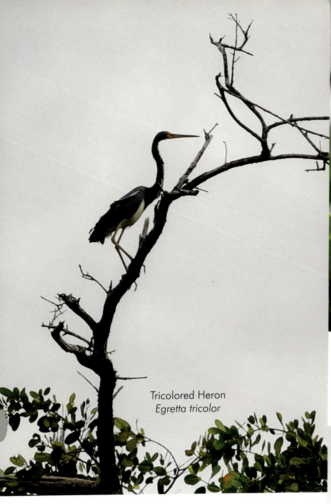

Tricolored Heron
*Egretta tricolor*

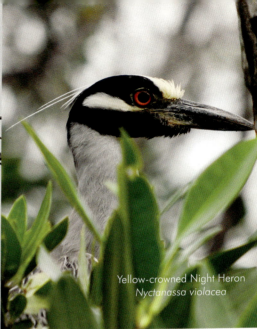

Yellow-crowned Night Heron
*Nyctanassa violacea*

Aquatic and many other birds find safe grounds in thick mangroves where they can hunt for food and build nests.

In the Tres Ríos Nature Park birds can be observed in their natural habitat. Smaller aquatic animals and insects that live in the roots and tree trunks sustain a significant population of different birds and their offspring each year.

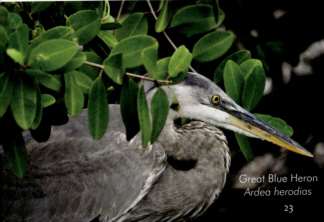

Great Blue Heron
*Ardea herodias*

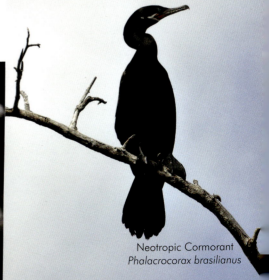

Neotropic Cormorant
*Phalacrocorax brasilianus*

# Bitter Orange

## Spanish Name: Naranja Agria
### Scientific Name: Citrus aurantium L.

9-10 fresh leaves of bitter orange were boiled in 3 glasses of water for 2 minutes, set to steep for 10 minutes, then one cup was taken before every meal for fever, diarrhea, and intestinal colic.

In cases of nervousness, hysteria, insomnia, and anxiety one small bunch of flowers was put in 3 glasses of boiling water for 20 minutes and one glass of this infusion was taken before meals.

To relieve high blood pressure 2-3 spoons of fresh juice were takren per day were taken for 10 days.

Juice from bitter orange mixed with water is good for kidney pain, it stimulates appetite, facilitates healing of internal hemorrhages and is a good general tonic.

For stomach pain an infusion of several leaves of bitter orange and oregano is made and taken only one time.

For many centuries the essential oil from the leaves of the bitter orange, called petit grain, was used as a remedy against depression.

Bitter orange comes from a citrus evergreen tree native to tropical Asia. It has served many ancient cultures for its medicinal effects and today the leaves, flowers, peel and juice of the fruit are used in numerous home remedies, bitter orange teas, tinctures, and extracts. Of particular value is the oil that is extracted from the peel. Both ripe and unripe fruit is used, although unripe bitter orange is more potent than when it is ripe.

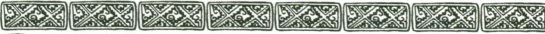

"Health and well-being can be achieved only by remaining centered in spirit, guarding against the squandering of energy, promoting the constant flow of qi and blood, maintaining harmonious balance of yin and yang, adapting to the changeing seasonal and yearly macrocosmic influences, and nourishing one's self preventively. This is the way to a long and happy life."
Huang Di, The Yellow Emperor

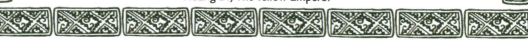

# trees of the forest

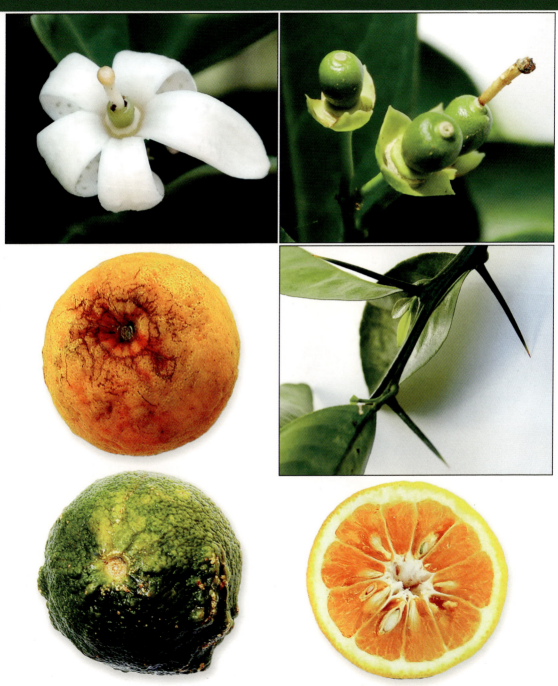

In Chinese medicine bitter orange is considered to be one of the strongest *chi* or *qi* moving herbs, with the power to help break up tumors. Bitter orange peel is safe in small amounts.

# Cacao
## Theobroma Cacao

All true chocolate comes from the ground seeds of the *Theobroma cacao*, a tropical tree that needs a lot of rain and humidity and grows very close to the equator. The cacao tree is believed to be native to Mesoamerica. The residue found in a pot dating to 400 BC suggests that the Maya may have been the first ones to make use of the wild cocoa beans, which then were cultivated extensively throughout the entire Classic period. The Mayas' appreciation for chocolate extended far beyond everyday indulgence; various recipes of the drink were used for religious and royal ceremonies and at weddings. This drink was indispensable to a good meal and its energy value was well known.

Criollo cacao pod

The Aztec civilization also held cacao in high regard, telling of the myth of *Quetzalcoatl*, the "Feathered Serpent" god, who was punished by the other gods for revealing the secret of cacao to humans. The very word 'cacao' comes from *cacahuatl,* a word in the Aztec language of *Nahuatl*. The Aztec chocolate was identical to the Mayan in basic preparation, but the Aztecs often added black pepper, vanilla beans, and the seed of a local tree called *achiote,* which dyed the drink bright red for use in rituals.

There are three main varieties: criollo, forastero y trinitario, besides some interesting local hybrids. Their prices and quality are highly variable. The most prized variety is the pure criollo characterized by white beans when fresh. It represents about 5% of all grown cacao.

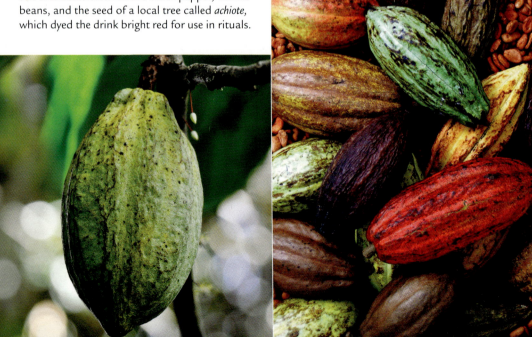

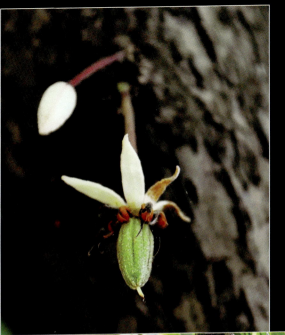

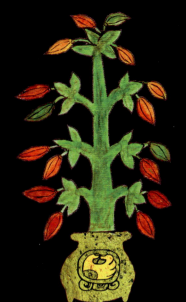

Left: Cacao flowers are pollinated by midges or ants.

Right: Ancient Mayan style drawing of a cacao plant.

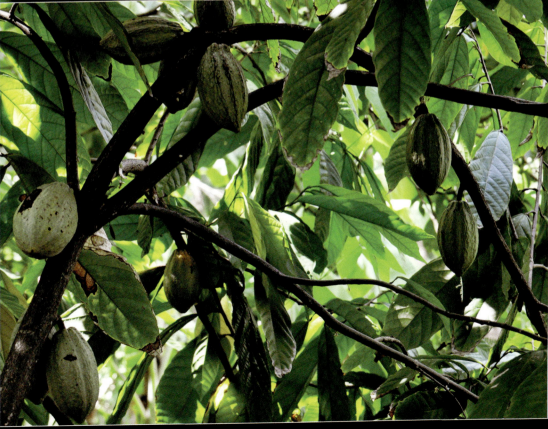

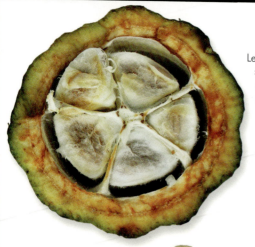

Left: Cross section of ripe cacao pod.

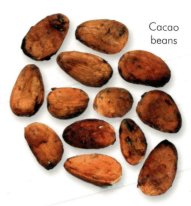

Cacao beans

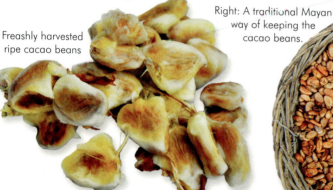

Freashly harvested ripe cacao beans

Right: A traditional Mayan way of keeping the cacao beans.

The fine tradition of Belgian chocolatiers meets the exquisite flavor and quality of the Mexican organically grown criollo cacao, resulting in a supreme quality. Below: Handmade pralines by ki'XOCOLATL.

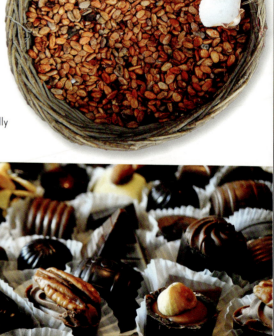

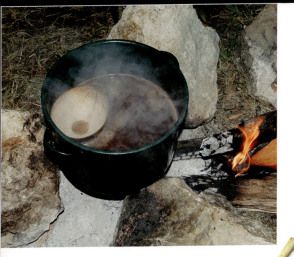

The drink *chocolatl* means bitter water, from *xococ* (bitter), and *atl* (water) and it traditionally was prepared only by the hands of the women during a long process. First the cacao beans were cleaned in water and dried in the sun, then toasted on a comal and ground several times in a mortar with a few grains of toasted corn. Then the paste was mixed with water, cooked over the fire and stirred with a *molinillo*, a frisk made of wood, until frothy. Aromatic spices such as vanilla, chile or honey were often added. This way of growing and drinking cacao spread to many areas of Mexico and Central America and is still practiced today.

*Chocolate de mesa* is chocolate ready to be prepared into a drink. There are many varieties, some infused with spices or enriched with nuts.

Cacao is a tonic. It stimulates the function of the nervous system and is an excellent remedy for weakness and physical exhaustion. Eating chocolate can improve your mood and bring anti-oxidants into your body.

"Certified Organic" defines a product grown and produced without chemicals that deplete the soil or damage the ecosystem. Organic and fair trade chocolate supports healthy farming and business practices.

Cacao is also believed to be very beneficial for the cardiovascular system.

Cacao butter is an excellent product used for cosmetic purposes. It nourishes dry and chapped skin overexposed to sun or cold. It is good to use in the making of natural ointments and salves.

*Molinillo*

Left: Dark chocolate bars by ki' XOCOLATL.

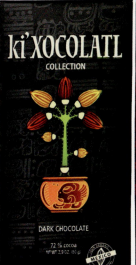
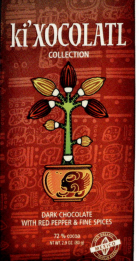

ki'XOCOLATL uses carefully selected organic criollo beans, which are roasted without having been previously washed in order to preserve the unique flavor of the criollo cacao. The beans are then refined until a fine paste is obtained, which based on the European tradition is then carefully blended for a minimum of twelve hours.

Eco-Museo del Cacao, the only museum of chocolate in Mexico, is located on Plantacion Tikul in the state of Yucatan, next to the archeological sites of Labna and Uxmal. Plantacion Tikul ia a sustainable project of growing organically red, white and other varieties of the criollo cacao. Located on over 200 acres this plantation combines the most advanced agricultural technology with traditional farming practices.

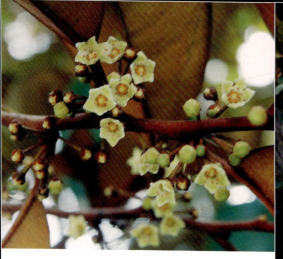

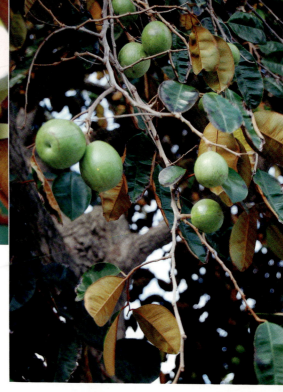

# Caimito
## Chrysophyllum cainito

Caimito is a tropical tree that reaches up to 20 m in height and has very beautiful foliage. The fruit is sold in local markets and is usually eaten fresh. The leaves in infusion with honey act as an expectorant. A poultice of leaves applied to bruises has a haemostatic effect. The bark has been used to treat diarrhea.

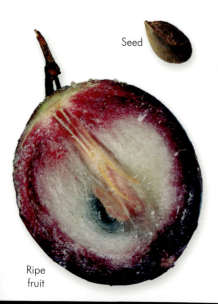

Seed

Ripe fruit

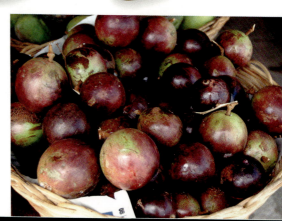

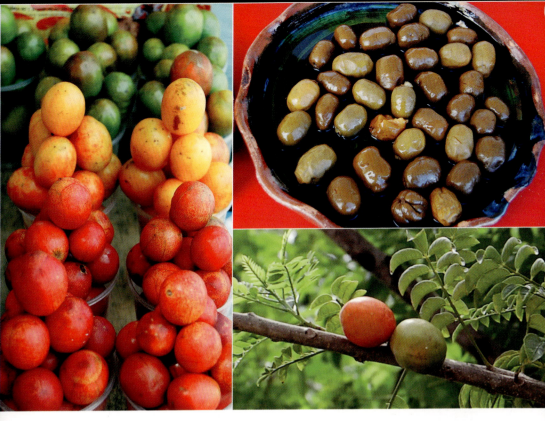

# Hog Plum
## Ciruela Jobo
### Spondias mombin

Mexican plum is native to the tropical Americas, it is a small tree distantly related to mango. Most of the varieties, of which there are about 20 just in the Yucatan Peninsula, have thick leathery skin and very little pulp. An infusion of flowers and bark is used traditionally for diarrhea, malaria fever, minor digestive disorders and as a contraceptive. A decoction of the bark and root is believed to have anti-septic properties. Wood fiber is good for papermaking.

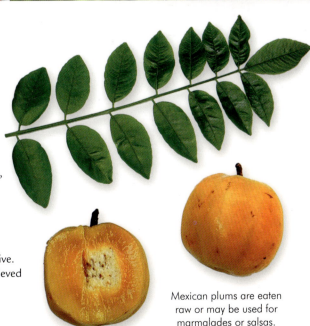

Mexican plums are eaten raw or may be used for marmalades or salsas.

SPANISH NAME: COCO
SCIENTIFIC NAME: COCOS NUCIFERA L.

# Coconut Tree

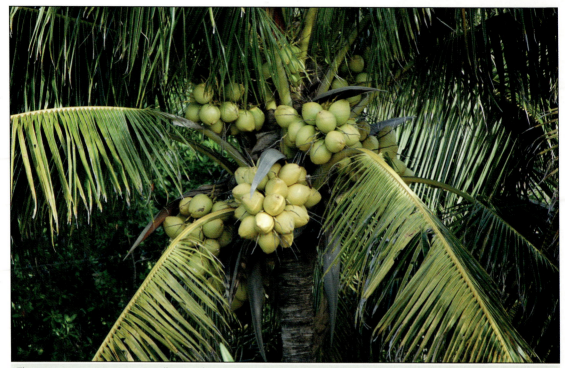

The coconut tree is common to all tropical countries. It likes sandy soil and in good conditions may live up to 100 years. Coconut tree is used for decorative purposes and when cultivated every part of it is used.

Coconut water from unripe coconuts is used fresh and is a popular drink rich in anti-oxidants. Depending on its size a coconut may contain from 300 ml to 1 l of liquid.

Coconut water is reccomended during fever, it purifies the blood and is a good liver and urinary system tonic.

Roots of the palm tree were used to prepare a mouth wash and to produce a fabric dye.

Coconut oil is very easily extracted by grating the pulp and boiling it. Coconut oil is excellent in ointments, lip balms and as a carrier oil for essential oils.

As a remedy against parasites, a blend of coconut liquid and pulp with a pinch of salt was taken on an empty stomach.

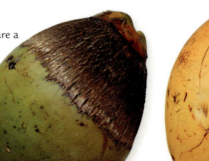
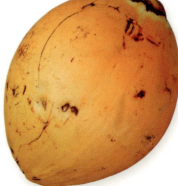

# trees of the forest

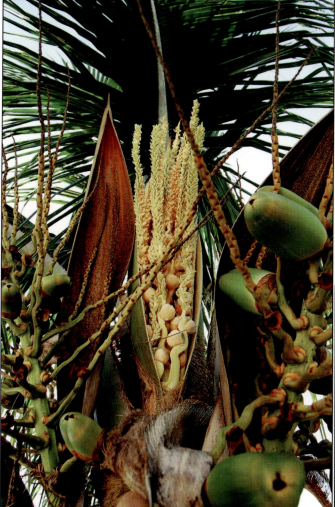

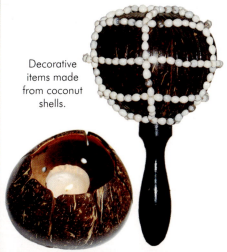

Decorative items made from coconut shells.

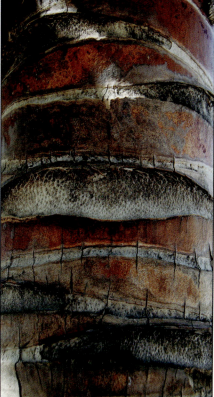

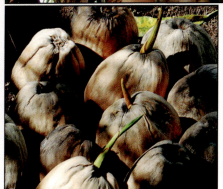

Above left: The palm tree flowers all year round.

Right: Trunk of a mature coconut palm.

Below left: Dry coconuts sprout if left on the ground.

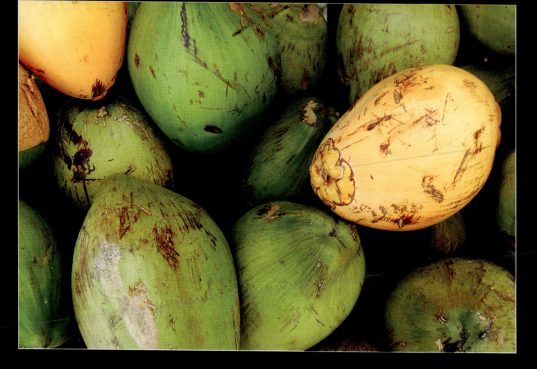

# Enjoy fresh coconut – a popular Mexican snack!
Coconut pulp contains high amounts of saturated fat and is low in sugar, high in proteins and zinc, iron and phosphorus.

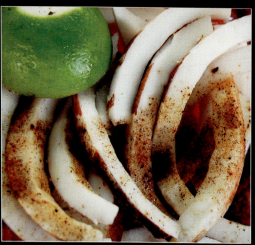

Coco strips with lime and chile habañero

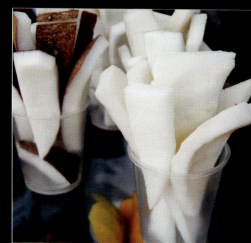

Chilled fresh coconut

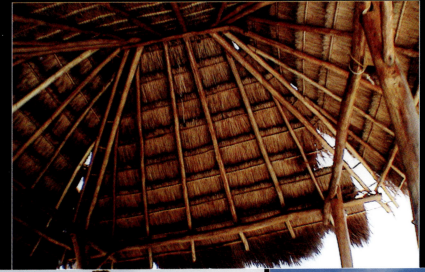

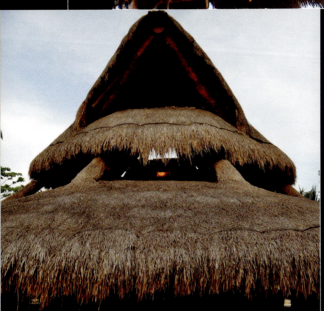

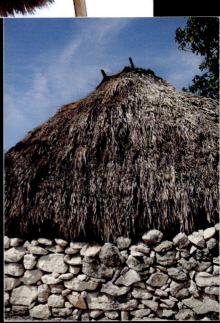

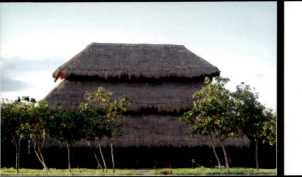

## Palapa roofs

The leaves of many different palm trees are woven into a variety of objects, from hats and baskets to hammocks, and are a universal roofing material. It is necessary to harvest the palm leaves in accordance with the Moon cycles in order for the roofing to last. Palm wood is a soft wood used in construction along with hard wood.

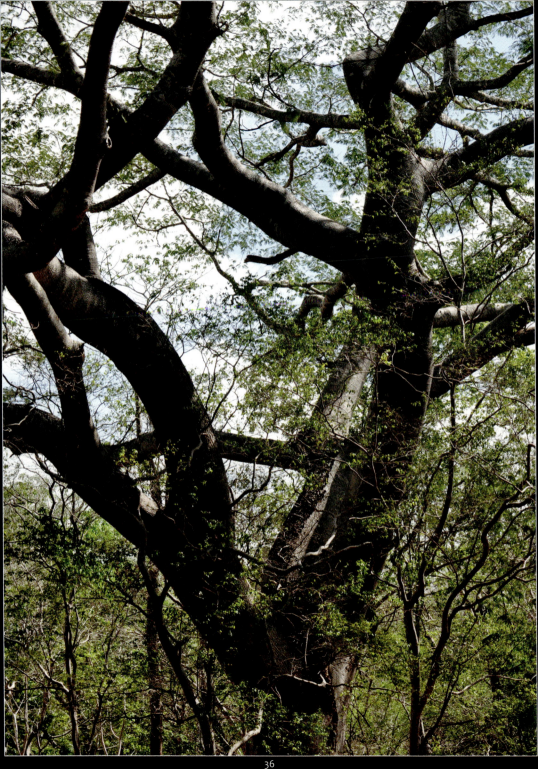

# Elephant Ear Tree
## Parota
### Enterolobium cyclocarpum

*Parota*, or *pich* in Mayan, is a very fast growing tree and one of the biggest in the forest, reaching up to 35-40 m in height and several m in diameter. Cultivated during the times of the ancient Mayan civilization, these trees are frequently found growing at archeological sites.

*Parota* wood is light and easy to carve and is used for mirror and door frames, decorative paneling and table tops for its beautiful variation of light to reddish-brown colors. The leaves have a high protein content and were used as food for the farm animals.

The fruit ripens almost one year later after the flowering occurs and usually generously covers the ground under the tree. *Parota* likes a lot of sun and is an excellent tree to provide shelter for people, cattle and other crops such as coffee or cacao. Clusters of small white flowers are favorite of small stingless bees.

The unripe green fruit of the tree was used in native cuisine. The sweet pulp surrounding the seed was also used. The seed is used for jewelry and crafts.

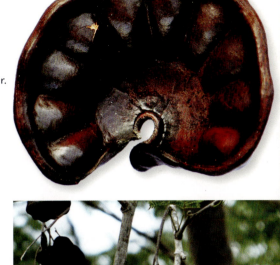
Fruit

Seeds

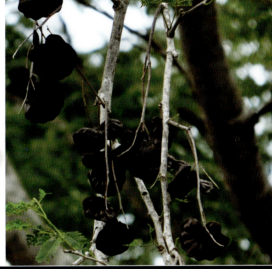

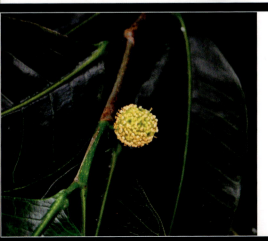

# Breadnut
## Ramón
### Brosimum alicastrum

Maya nut has been cultivated in Central America for thousands of years and was one of the original native trees in the Mayan forest. The seed of the fruit was used cooked, roasted or dried in the sun and ground into flour. It is very nutritious, high in fiber, vitamins A, C, iron, zinc, potassium, calcium and folic acid. Maya nut has a high protein content and a very pleasant flavor when roasted. The fruit ripens in spring and is collected from the ground.

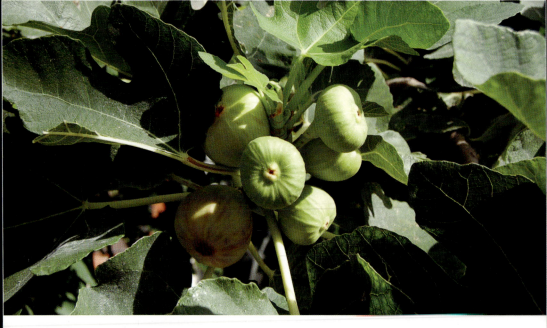

# Fig Tree
## Higuera
### Ficus carica L.

The fig tree is believed to have originated in Asia, where it has been found in excavations dating back to 5000 BC. In his writings Pliny mentions 29 different varieties of figs known in his time. While everywhere else fig trees grow tall, sometimes reaching the height of 30 m, in the Yucatan they are mostly found as tall shrubs due to high humidity. Figs are distant relatives of mulberry and breadnut. Sycamore fig, another member of the family, is a favorite fruit in Egypt and Syria.

Figs are delicious fresh or dry and have a very high nutritional value. In some countries ripe fruit is used to make a type of sweet wine.

In traditional medicine figs have been used for their mild laxative effect. Warm decoctions of figs are used as a remedy for catarrhs and sore throat.

Figs roasted over the fire and cut in halves were applied to boils and abscesses in biblical times.

Milky resin from the stems is used as a remedy to remove warts.

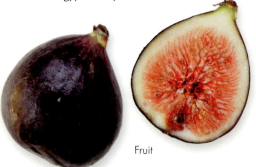

Fruit

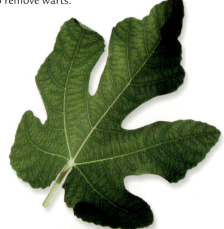

# Serret
## Nance
### Byrsonima crassifolia

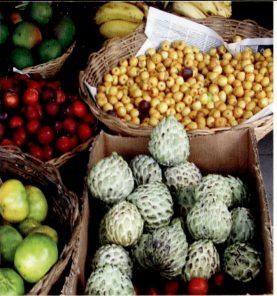

Serret trees are very common in tropical America. They are used as ornamental items and also cultivated for the small, yellow fruit that they bare. The trees grow very slowly, but overtime may reach the height of 20 m.

Serret fruit has a strong scent and may be eaten raw or made into a dessert. The dessert prepared with the addition of honey and flour and known as pesada de nance is quite popular in Central American countries. The fruits are also made into dulce de nance, a candy prepared with the fruit cooked in sugar and water.

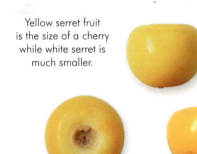

Yellow serret fruit is the size of a cherry while white serret is much smaller.

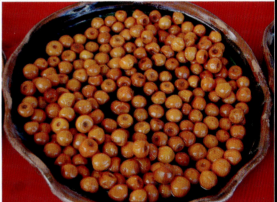

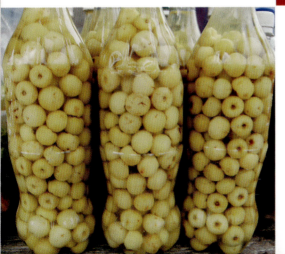

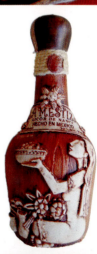

Above right: Serret in sweet syrup.

Left: White serret pickled with chile.

Right: Serret liquor, a specialty of the Yucatan Peninsula.

# Geiger Tree

## Spanish Name: Ciricote
### Scientific Name: Cordia dodecandra A.

Ciricote bark and wood boiled in a decoction is used for common colds, diarrhea, dysentery and chills.

Flowers in infusion act as an expectorant and are more beneficial when combined with other plants with similar properties, such as papaya flowers and avocado or mango leaves.

In folk medicine a decoction of geiger tree flowers and fruit was used to alleviate minor respiratory conditions, catarrhs, bronchitis and respiratory congestion. The decoction was prepared with 40 g of fruit and flowers cooked slowly in 1.5 l of water. When cooled off, 2-3 tbsp. were taken throughout the day, sometimes with lime and honey.

The tree sap is used on wounds.

A poultice made of fresh leaves may be applied for headaches or on strains for temporary relief.

The *ciricote* is a tall and fast growing tree that tolerates salty soil very well and is found close to the coastline throughout the Yucatan Peninsula. When *ciricote* grows further away from the sea it can become very tall, up to 10 m in height. It is easily recognized because of the clusters of bright orange flowers. The fruit is prepared in syrup or eaten fresh when ripe.

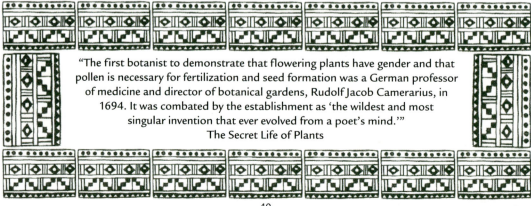

"The first botanist to demonstrate that flowering plants have gender and that pollen is necessary for fertilization and seed formation was a German professor of medicine and director of botanical gardens, Rudolf Jacob Camerarius, in 1694. It was combated by the establishment as 'the wildest and most singular invention that ever evolved from a poet's mind.'"
The Secret Life of Plants

# trees of the forest

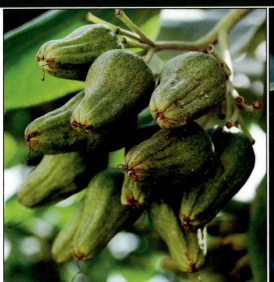

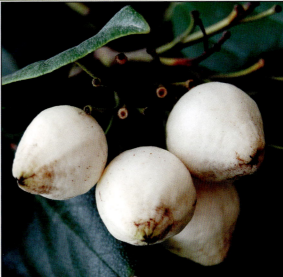

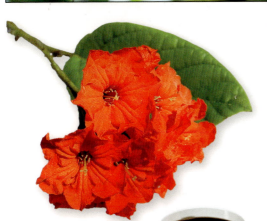

Cough syrup could be made by cooking fruit and flowers for about 30 minutes in the double boiler. Strain well, keep refrigerated, and take one table spoon before meals.

*Ciricote* fruit cooked in honey or cane sugar in syrup is a tasty local treat.

# Guava

### Spanish Name: Guayaba
Scientific Name: Psidium guajava L.

The *guayava* is a common tree in the tropics, reaching up to 10 m in height. *Guayava* fruit is very high in vitamin C, vitamin A and is also a good source of pectin. The leaves of *guayava* possess essential oil and tannin, and are rich in flavonoids, in particular quercetin, all known for their anti-bacterial properties.

*Guayava* roots, leaves, bark and fruit have been used in traditional medicine as a remedy for digestive infections, intestinal colic and for its general anti-inflammatory effect. 30 g of leaves, bark and root are boiled in 1 l of water for 30 minutes after which one cup is taken 3 times a day. The bark is known to have been a remedy for dysentery.

A few fresh *guayava* leaves are a good addition to an herbal infusion. It helps to clear out coughs, sore throat and minor respiratory congestion. An avocado leaf, 2-3 papaya flowers, *guayava* leaf, bitter orange leaf, a slice of ginger and a little honey make a wonderful infusion for minor colds and congestion.

In case of toothache leaves may be chewed, but not swallowed, to provide a temporary relief. Leaf decoction may serve as a mouth rinse for oral ulcers and inflamed gums.

A poultice made of fresh leaves may be applied on minor wounds, ulcers and rheumatic spots.

To calm itching rash or to dry up hives, heat rash, chicken pox or scarlet fever, use mashed leaves mixed in water as a rinse or a bath.

Thick, rich guava paste and guava jelly are popular in Central and South America.

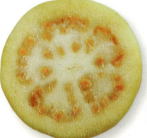

The fruit is very flavorful and has very small, hard, yellow seeds that are strained when drinks are made.

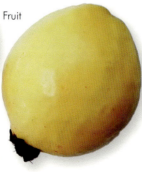

Fruit

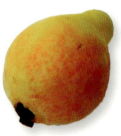

# trees of the forest

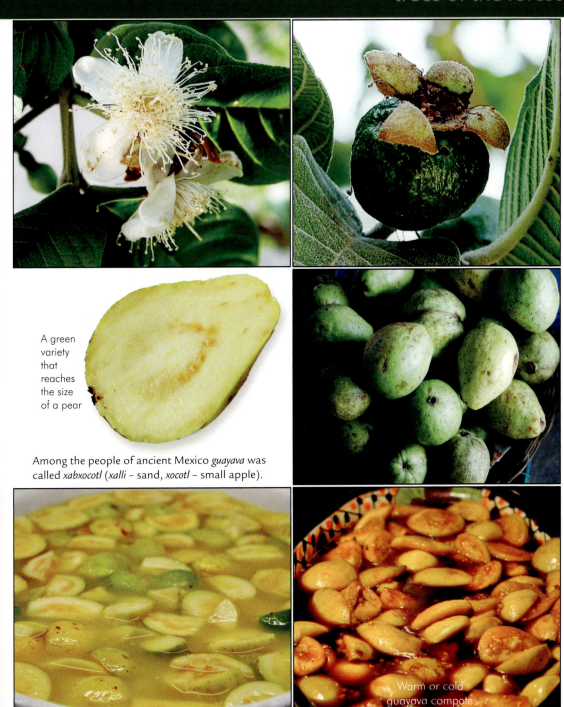

A green variety that reaches the size of a pear

Among the people of ancient Mexico *guayava* was called *xabxocotl* (*xalli* – sand, *xocotl* – small apple).

Warm or cold guayava compote

# Huaya
## Mamoncillo
### Melicoccus bijugatus

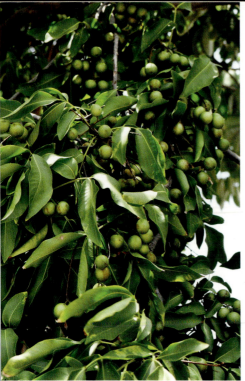

The huaya is a large tropical tree native to the American continents. The fruit, similar to lychee, ripens in summer and is sold in bunches at farmer's markets.

The fruit is eaten without the skin. The juice was used as a fabric dye; it produces a nice deep brown color. Each fruit has a seed that can be roasted and eaten as well.

The huaya has small, green fragrant flowers. It blossoms from the branch tips in the onset of the rainy season.

The huaya tree is also commonly planted along roadsides as an ornamental tree.

This fruit can be sweet or sour. In the southern areas of Mexico it is generally eaten with chili powder, salt, and lime. The sweet varieties are served without any condiments.

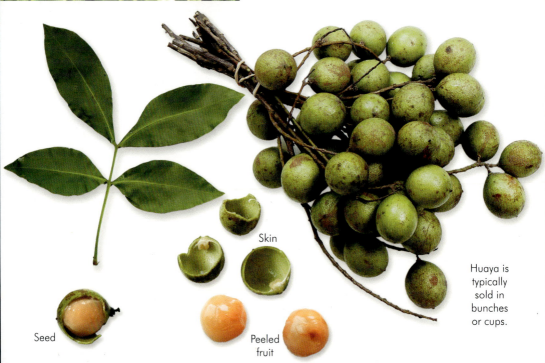

Seed

Skin

Peeled fruit

Huaya is typically sold in bunches or cups.

# Custard Apple
## Tejocote
### Crataegus mexicana

The custard apple is a bush which sometimes grows up to 6 m tall. It has thorns and produces small white flowers. All parts of the plant are used medicinally.

The root is believed to have diuretic properties and in herbal medicine is used to detox and stimulate the kidneys. Traditionally 15 g of the root were cooked in 200 g of water until half of the liquid boiled out and the decoction was taken in small amounts 2-3 times a day. The same decoction was used for inflammations related to the urinary system.

The fruit has a very delicious flavor and is very beneficial for respiratory conditions, the circulatory system and blood vessels.
Try it in the following infusion:

1 *guayava*

2 *tejocote*
2-3 dry jamaica flowers

a rind of ginger

add lime and honey to your taste

# Bay Cedar
## Guásimo
### Guazuma ulmifolia

Bay cedar trees may grow very tall. They are very common in the Yucatan Peninsula. Native bees like its small yellow flowers. The seeds are abundant and may be used as food for domestic animals. The tough, fibrous bark and young stems are used to make rope and twine. The wood is easy to work and very durable.

A beverage of crushed seeds soaked in water is used to treat diarrhea, dysentery, colds and coughs. It has diuretic and astringent properties.

Seeds

# Mamey

## Spanish Name: Mamey
### Scientific Name: Mammeya americana

The pulp of the fruit is delicate and sweet and is a good tonic for the digestive system.

A decoction of the bark is used as a rinse for skin infections and irritations.

The resin that comes out of mamey trunk mixed with oil was applied to cracked skin. It is also very efective to rid animals of ticks and fleas.

Powdered seeds applied externally is a remedy for skin parasites.

Dried and powdered unripe fruit has insecticide properties.

Infusion of fresh or dry leaves has been used by traditional healers as a quinine substitute for malaria and dengue fever.

The mamey is a tree that is very common in Mexico and is almost unknown outside of the American continents. It is related to mangosteen. The mamey is a delicate tree that likes rich and dry soil. The trunk of the tree may reach up to 1 m in diameter. The foliage is very beautiful and the color and shape of the leaves make it easy to recognize.

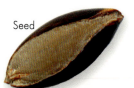
Seed

The fruit is consumed fresh, as an addition to smoothies or made into ice cream. A popular desert is mamey fruit cut in small cubes, soaked in a small amount of sweet red wine and honey and served chilled.

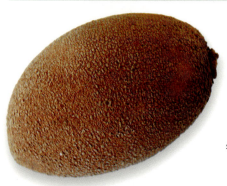

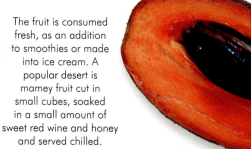

# trees of the forest

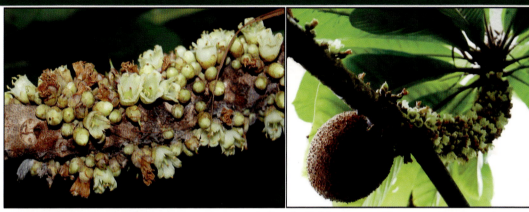

Small fragrant mamey flowers appear during and after the fruiting season. They grow directly on the stem.

## Grosella

The *grosella* is a fruit that grows on the tree and is very common throughout the Yucatan Peninsula. It is not related to European currants.

Mexican *grosella* has a very tart and sour taste and is high in fiber and vitamin C. It is most commonly served with lime and chile.

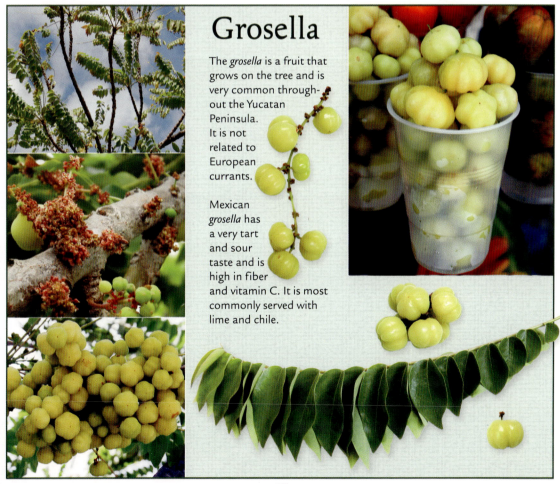

# Mangrove, Red

**Spanish Name:** Mangle Rojo
**Scientific Names:** Rhizophora mangle L.

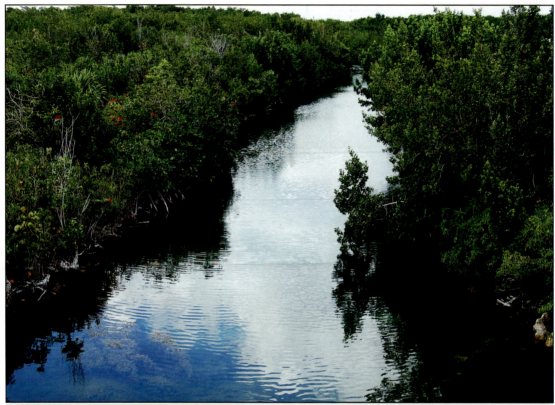

Mangrove trees are typical for the tropical coastlines and have a similar distribution as coral reefs. On the Mexican Caribbean coast the 3 most common types of mangrove trees are the black, the white and the red mangroves, which grow very close to the sea line. Red mangroves grow up to 5 m in height and form islands of thick bushes with the root system spread below the water surface. Birds, lizards, small mammals, alligators and a variety of sea animals live in the mangroves.

Red mangroves were used in folk medicine for centuries for a wide range of ailments. The part used medicinally is the bark. It is better to let crushed red mangrove bark stand in cold water for 2 hours before preparation.

For inflammation of the bile canals or gall bladder a decoction of 6 g of bark for 100 g of water is taken on empty stomach for 3 days.

Red mangrove has astringent qualities and externally a decoction of the bark may be used as a rinse for acne or chickenpox.

Red mangrove bark was used as a tonic for the digestive system.

Red mangrove decoctions were used for leprosy in a bath.

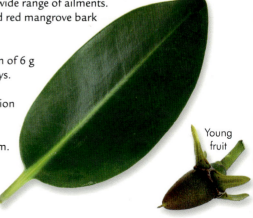

Young fruit

# trees of the forest

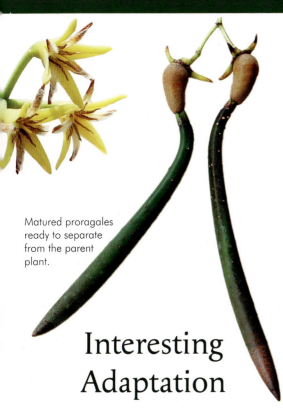

Matured proragales ready to separate from the parent plant.

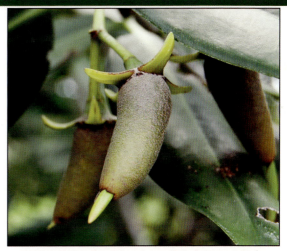

The fruit, or proragale, is an embryo of a new plant; it falls off into the water when mature and can float for over 6 months until it attaches its root system in a permanent location.

## Interesting Adaptation

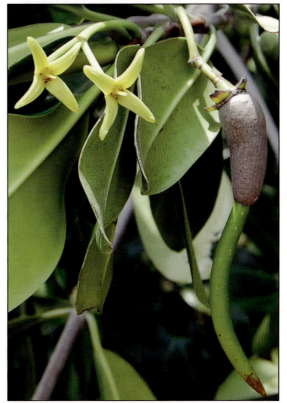

Growing in salty coastal soils, mangrove trees limit the amount of moisture that they lose through their leaves by adjusting the openings of small pores. The trees also turn their leaves to avoid the burning midday sun and reduce evaporation through the leaf surface.

Mangrove trees evolved a unique way to support the survival of new plants. The seeds of red mangroves germinate while still on the parent tree through the fruit and produce their own food via photosynthesis. Mature propagales fall into the water to be transported sometimes very far away. When ready to root, propagales are able to float vertically rather than horizontally due to a change in the density that occurrs in preparation for permanent rooting. If the rooting fails the density goes back to normal allowing the propagales to float easily in a horizontal position again.

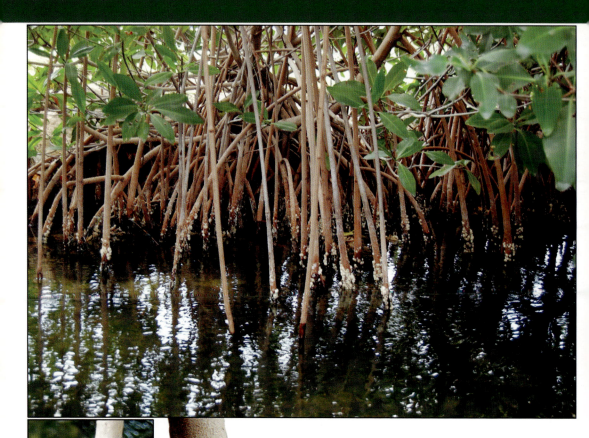

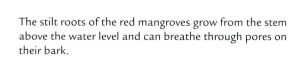

The stilt roots of the red mangroves grow from the stem above the water level and can breathe through pores on their bark.

Red mangroves exclude salt by having rather impermeable roots which act as an efficient filtration mechanism to separate sodium salts from the rest of the plant.

During extreme storms and hurricanes mangrove forests protect coastal areas by limiting damage from the waves, currents and winds.

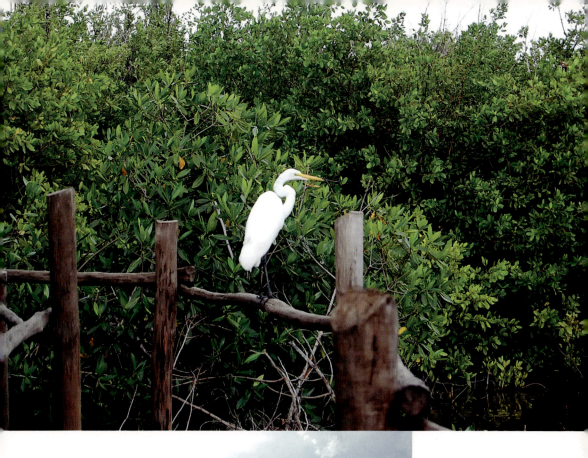

Above: Mangroves host a wide variety of birds.

Right: Dried mangrove trees are used as part of the landscape design.

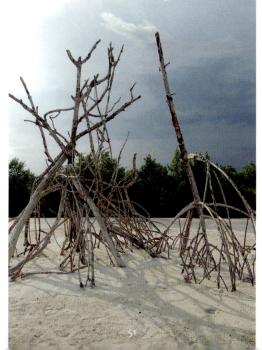

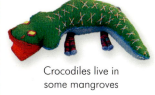

Crocodiles live in some mangroves

# Native Hardwood    Maderas Indigenas

There are several types of very beautiful hardwood trees in the tropical forest, which when harvested properly may be used for construction, arts or crafts and last for many hundreds of years. During the dry season forest fires result in many old fallen trees. They are cut and handled by experienced carpenters to be turned into very valuable and attractive pieces.

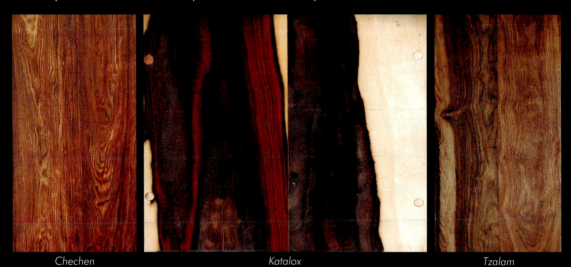

Chechen    Katalox    Tzalam

The *chechen* tree has bright colored wood ranging from amber to bright brown. It is a very hard and dense wood, a very popular material in the Yucatan Peninsula due to its high resistance to rotting. After the bark and resin is removed, it is safe to handle and is fashioned into cabinets and furniture.

*Katalox*, or *Swartzia cubensis,* is the most beautiful of local woods, with vibrant color variations. *Katalox* wood is very hard and difficult to work.

*Tsalam*, or *Lysiloma bahamensis,* is medium brown, smooth and very pleasant to touch. This prized wood is used to create beautiful and lasting pieces of furniture and interior design.

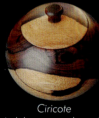

Ciricote
A delicate wood mostly used for arts and crafts.

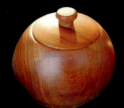

Banyan Tree

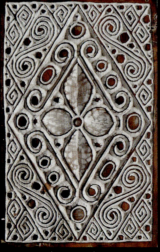

Modern woodcarving

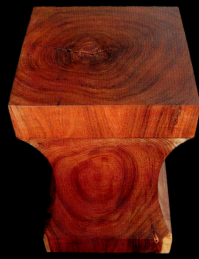

Zapote Blanco

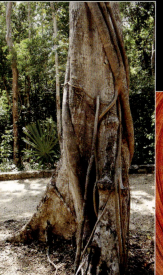
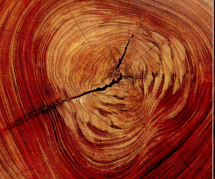

Left: There are some big trees like *zapote, ramon* or ceiba that develop a buttress which helps them to remain in an upright position when the layer of soil is thin or soft.

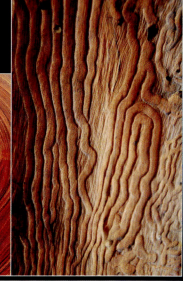

# Woodworking and woodcarving

The Maya were experienced boat builders and had a constant traffic that used river and sea, reaching as far north as present day Tampico in the Panuco River and south to Nicaragua and Panama. The length and complexity of the traveling routes suggests that the boats were very sturdy and an important means of transportation and trade. *Cayucos* had flat bottoms and could carry a lot of merchandise such as jade, feathers, salt, honey, vegetable inks, obsidian tools, medicinal herbs, dry chiles, tree resin and grinding stones.

Canoes and *cayucos* were built from one piece of wood, hollowed out by fire and sealed by resin.

Tulum, a main Mayan seaport and trade center, was famous for its canoe makers, some reached the length of 30 m and could hold up to 50 people.

Woodcarving remains a popular craft at present time. Right: An elaborate Mayan style carving typical for the Yucatan Peninsula.

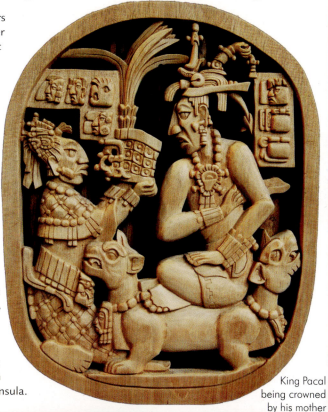

King Pacal being crowned by his mother

# Sapodilla Tree
## Chicozapote
### Manilkara zapota

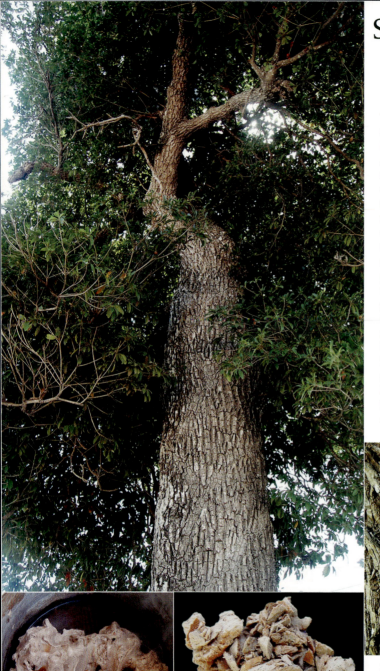

The sapodilla tree is one of the most common in the Yucatan Peninsula. It is known as the *Arbol del Chicle,* or Chewing Gum Tree, because of its sticky white sap, or *chicle*. Sapodilla trees are some of the tallest in the tropical forests, growing up to 80 m. A tree takes 20 years to mature before it can be tapped for chicle. The *Chicleros,* people who collected the resin, tap the trees once every 7-8 years giving them time to recover from the deep cuts made in the bark. The resin flows best between July and December. Sapodilla wood is very durable and is used for supporting beams in construction. The bark of the sapodilla tree is very rich in tannin.

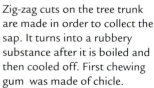

Zig-zag cuts on the tree trunk are made in order to collect the sap. It turns into a rubbery substance after it is boiled and then cooled off. First chewing gum was made of chicle.

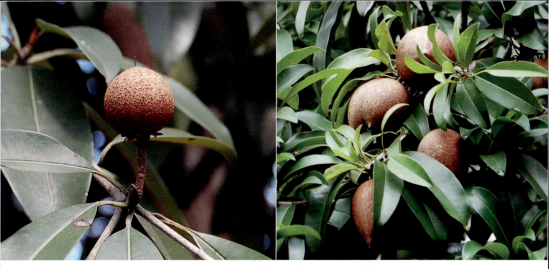

Sapodilla trees may yield fruit twice a year. The soft, light brown fruit matures when picked. It has a delicate and pleasant taste.

Old yellow leaves were traditionally used for colds and cough. Green leaves were believed to be a good remedy for diarrhea, hardened arteries and to regulate blood pressure.

Crushed seeds are used as a remedy for kidney stones. An alcohol extract made with the seeds was used in very small amounts before meals to calm the nerves, for insomnia or headache.

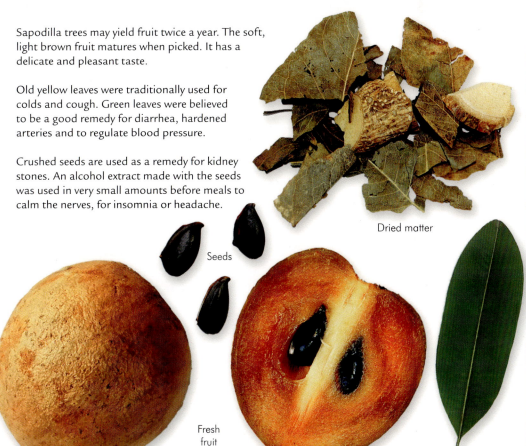

Dried matter

Seeds

Fresh fruit

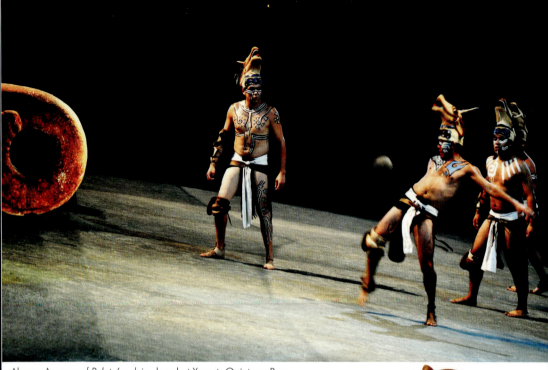

Above: A game of *Pok ta' pok* is played at Xcaret, Quintana Roo.

# The Mayan Ball Game Pok ta' pok

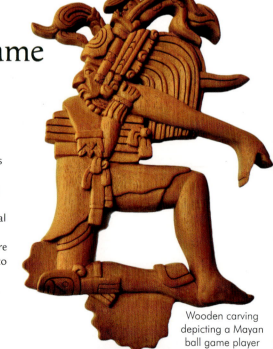

Possibly the first team sport practiced by man, *pok ta' pok* was a game practiced in several parts of Mesoamerica and there were ball courts in almost all Mayan cities. Most were rectangular, with a flat playing surface about 30-50 m long and 10-20 m wide, with either sloping or vertical walls and two big stone hoops on both sides. Two teams competed. We know that hands were not permitted and the object of the game was to get the ball through the stone hoop. It was propelled with the hips, shoulders or forearms. Elaborate rituals accompanied these contests.

Wooden carving depicting a Mayan ball game player

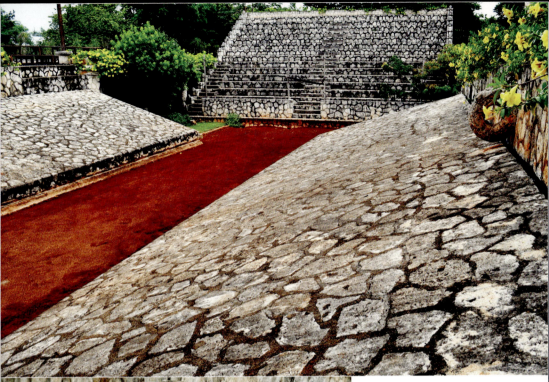

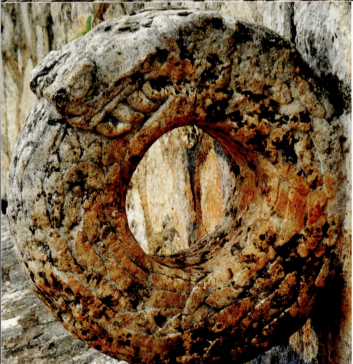

The ball game is believed to have been invented by the Olmecs around 3000 BC. A specially built court was called tlachco. In the *Popol Vuh* myth the Hero Twins *Hun Hunahpu* and *Xbalanque* beat the lords of the underworld in a ball game.

The ball was solid rubber, possibly made of *chicle* resin, 4 kg in weight and about 25 cm in diameter.

Bets were placed and tributes were offered to be taken by the winners after the game. Villages that supported their teams brought what they harvested or produced to be offered as a tribute.

**Spanish Name: Palmera Chit**
Scientific Name: Serenoa repens

# Saw Palmetto

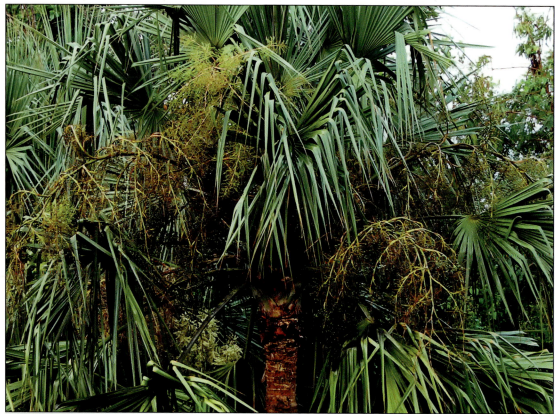

Saw palmetto is another palm tree very widely spread in the south east of Mexico. It may grow to 15-20 m in height, while the trunk is not more than 20-30 cm wide. It has round leaves up to 1-1.5 m in diameter. Palmera Chit is found in coastal forests and close to the sea, growing in the dunes or close to mangroves. It is an endangered variety that grows very slowly.

A decoction of berries used as a hair rinse is said to prevent hair loss.

Traditionally berries were believed to have expectorant and an antiseptic properties and to be a good mild sedative, and very beneficial for the digestive system.

At present time saw palmetto berries are used mainly for conditions associated with enlarged or inflamed prostate gland. In general the berries are a very good tonic for the reproductive and urinary systems of women and men because it helps to maintain hormonal balance.

In infusion fresh or dry berries may be used as a remedy for cough and other mild respiratory conditions.

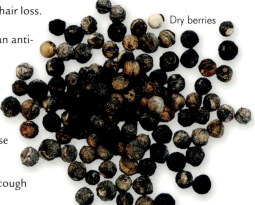

Dry berries

# trees of the forest

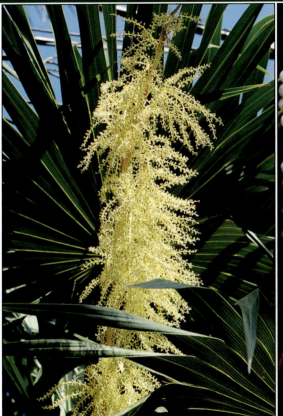

Palmera chit flowers are abundant with pollen.

Fresh fruit is 5 mm to 1 cm in diameter and is edible.

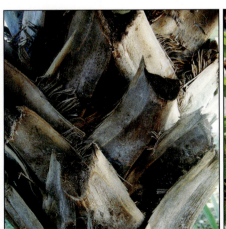 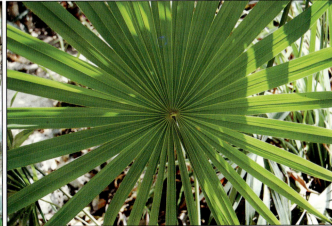

Fibers and leaves are widely used in crafts and rural construction.

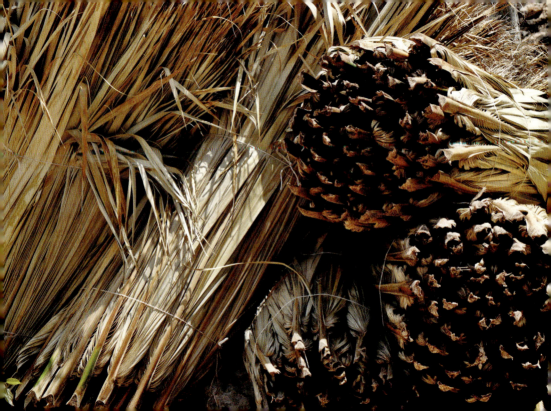

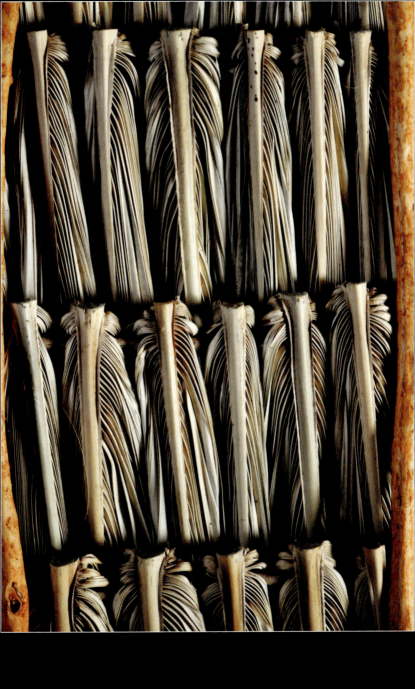

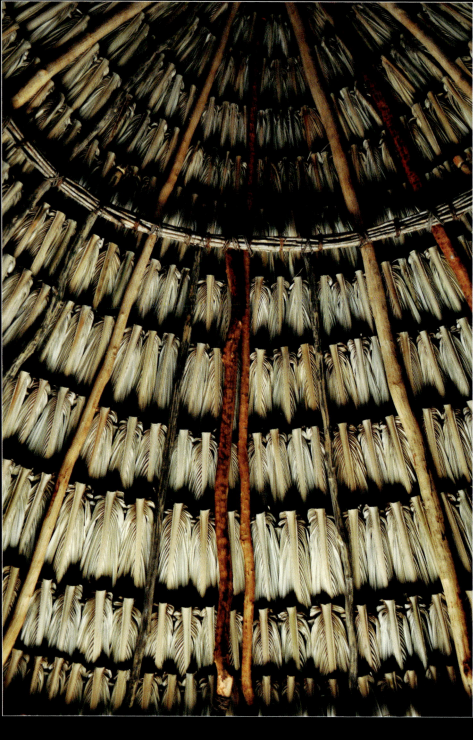

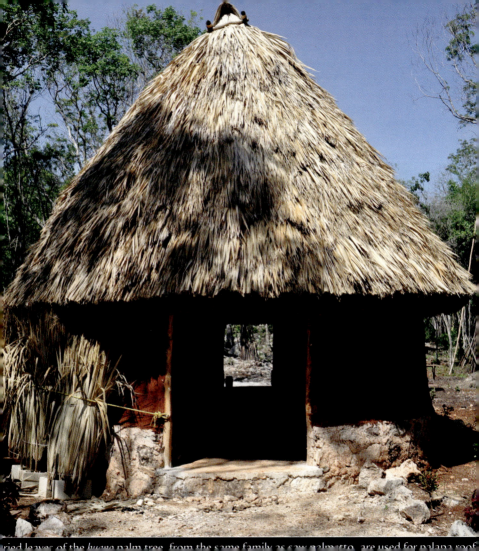

# Soursop

## Spanish Name: Guanabana
### Scientific Name: Annona muricata

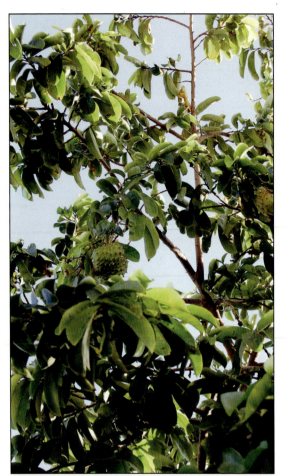

Soursop is a medium sized tree believed to have originated in the American continents. Like its relatives, anona and cherimoya, it thrives in the sun, humidity and high temperatures and is now very common to other tropical countries. There are about 60 species of the *Annona* family, soursop is the only one that is grown commercially and can be found outside of Mexico. The fruit may weigh from 200 g to 1.5 kg. It has a creamy pulp with a delicious flavor.

The bark of the *guanabana* tree made into infusion is a good remedy for asthma.

The juice from fresh fruit is effective against dysentery. When mixed with honey it also serves as a relief for fevers and excessive bile flow.

A decoction of fresh leaves helps in cases of diarrhea.

To provide relief for mild respiratory difficulties young leaves of *guanabana* are combined with the leaves of bull hoof, avocado, and mango in a decoction and taken in small servings during the entire day.

Leaves applied locally as a poultice have anti-inflammatory effect in case of mumps.

The flowers are pectoral and may be used in infusion for bronchial colds.

Leaves in infusion are used for insomnia.

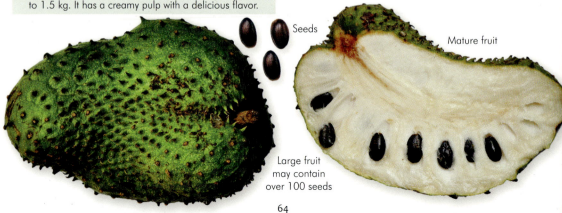

Seeds

Mature fruit

Large fruit may contain over 100 seeds

# trees of the forest

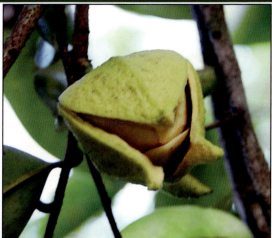

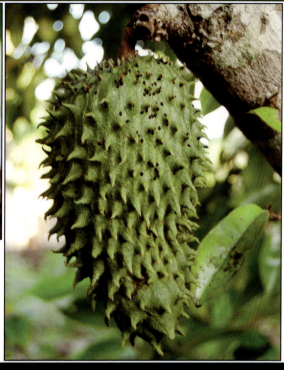

*Guanabana* fruit is very rich in carbohydrates, vitamins C, B1, B2 and phosphorus. *Guanabanas* that are not well ripened may be cooked as a vegetable.

**When processed, care needs to be taken to remove all the seeds because of their slight toxicity.**

## Guanabana and Camote

This recipe originated in Tabasco, where *camote, guanabana* and cane sugar are cooked together, spooned into corn husks, tied up and served as a sweet tamale for snacks or dessert.

---

Cook 3 orange yams in water with a few blades of lemongrass until very soft, mash until smooth, combine with ½ *guanabana* cleaned of skin, seeds and mashed, a pinch of salt and a few drops of honey. Squeeze juice of one lime, combine with 6 tbsp. of melted butter. Serve as a side dish or a warm dip.

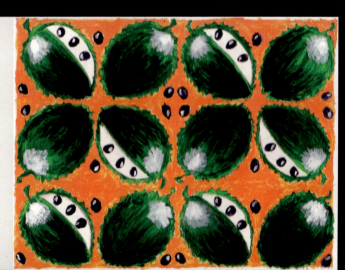

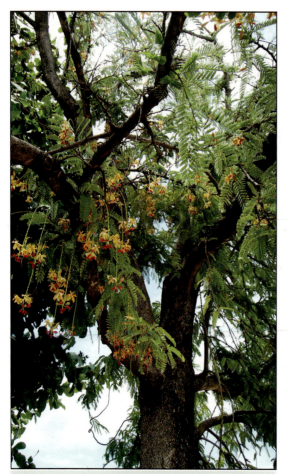

# Tamarind

## Spanish Name: Tamarindo
Scientific Name: Tamarindus indica L.

The leaves prepared as herbal tea reduce malaria fever.

Tamarind pulp is tasty on its own or made into a drink in combination with lime juice, honey, dates and spices. It is refreshing and promotes good digestion.

A decoction of 8 g of leaves in 100 ml of water gets rid of intestinal parasites and is beneficial in cases of dysentery.

Crushed seeds have been used as a remedy for diabetes.

Tamarind leaves and flowers, dried or boiled, are used as poultices for swollen joints, sprains and boils.

Locally the pulp is applied on inflammations and is used in a gargle for sore throat. Warmed pulp mixed with salt is a remedy for rheumatism.

The pulp is said to aid the restoration of sensation in cases of paralysis.

The tamarind is a slow growing evergreen tree native to Africa and common in the tropics and if planted in favorable conditions can reach up to 20 m. The fruit is a brown irregularly shaped pod with seeds embedded in the pulp. The pulp has a sweet and sour taste and it is high in both acid and sugar. The pods mature on the tree for about 6 months. When fully ripe the moisture content is reduced by up to 20%. It is very rich in vitamin B and high in calcium. The medicinal uses of tamarind are numerous.

"The source of vitality is the diet."
Huang Di, The Yellow Emperor

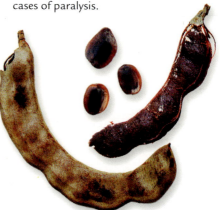

# trees of the forest

Tamarind pods may contain from one to a dozen seeds all enveloped in a thin brown membrane embedded in sticky pulp. To use the pulp the seeds and skin have to be removed, usually by adding water and straining. New plants are propagated from the seeds.

Tamarind pulp may be eaten fresh or prepared as a cooling drink. It is also used to flavor preserves, made into chutney and is a main flavor in Pad Thai.

Young leaves and very young seedlings and flowers may be cooked and eaten as greens or used in a curry as it is common in India. They also may be added to soups and the flowers used as an ingredient in salads.

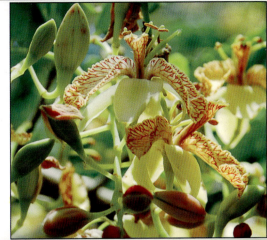

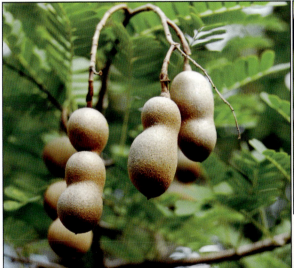

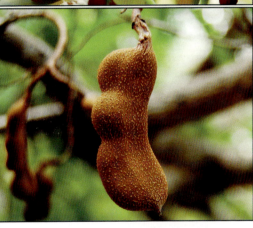

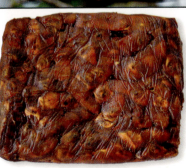

Tamarind pulp cleaned of skin and fiber is sold with seeds in it.

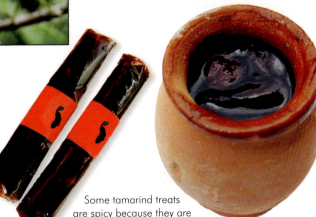

Some tamarind treats are spicy because they are made with the addition of chile.

# Tropical Almond

## Spanish Name: Almendro Tropical
### Scientific Name: Terminalia catappa L.

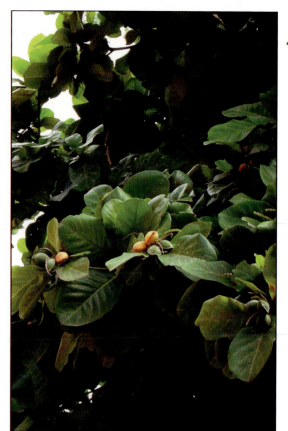

Tropical almond is a large tropical tree that originated in Asia and spread to most tropical countries. It is very common in the Yucatan Peninsula, having adapted well to salty soil. It grows in small inland towns and along the beaches, reaching the height of 25-30 m. Tropical almond tolerates the dry season very well, even though it likes well irrigated soil. Tropical almond can be used as an ornamental plant and grown in a flower pot, in which case its growth can be controlled.

There are two main varieties of almonds: sweet and bitter. While the sweet ones are grown commercially and the oil that is extracted from them is used in the food and cosmetic industries, some species of bitter almond contain very poisonous chemicals.

Oil of the bitter almond is a particularly strong poison.

Nuts of the tropical almond are not used for human consumption. Aerial parts have been used in traditional medicine and are believed to have anti-bacterial properties.

The leaves of the sweet almond used medicinally differ in their qualities depending on the stage of maturity: thus green, red and yellow leaves are used to treat different conditions.

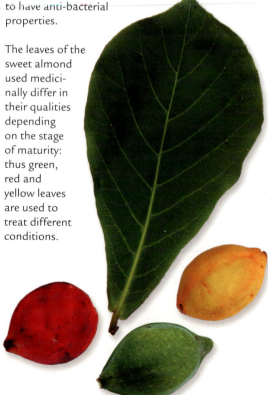

The fruit has a nut that is a favorite of squirrels and other small animals.

> "The magnet is a perfect expression of the basic principle of governing life: electricity and magnetism. These two principles rule everything. The human, which is a living magnet, has an electromagnetic field called the aura, which is composed of an electric and magnetic principle. Physical pain, discomfort and disease come from an imbalance of these two principles."
> The Divine Doctor, Joseph Michael Levry

# trees of the forest

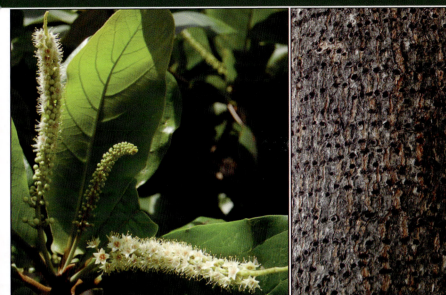

Tropical almond is a favorite of woodpeckers who leave rings of dots on the trunk (above right).

## Breadfruit
### Castaña
#### Artocarpus camansi

Native to New Guinea, breadfruit grows in the Yucatan Peninsula up to 10-15 m in height and yeilds about 700 fruits per season when fully mature. The white-yellow pulp has a pleasant taste. The seeds are high in protein and low in fat.

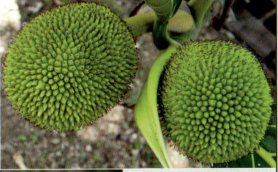

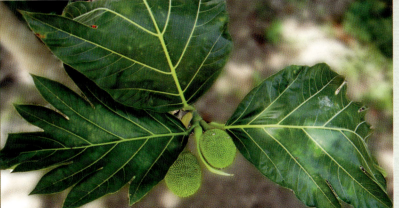

In traditional Mayan cooking the seed contained within the fruit was ground up and made into *masa*, or thick dough, for making *tortillas*. *Tortillas* were also made from the nut of the ramon tree and the coconut.

SPANISH NAME: GUARUMBO
SCIENTIFIC NAME: CECROPIA PELTATA L.

# Trumpet Tree

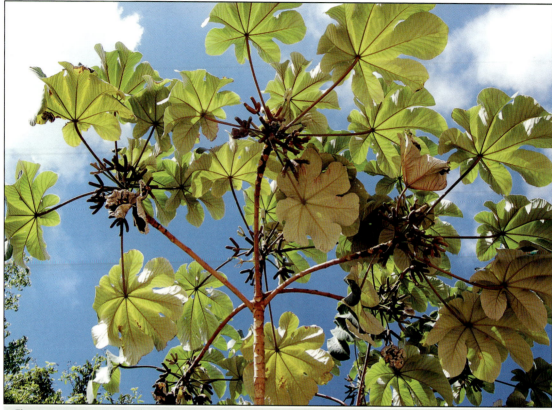

The trumpet tree is a tropical tree abundant in Mexican forests that reaches 20-25 m in height. It is usually among the first trees to appear on disturbed land, growing very fast and creating cover for less resistant plants. The seeds of the trumpet tree may remain dormant for about ten years, but will germinate as soon as they are exposed to sunlight. This is a pioneer plant that grows in sunny sites. Its large leaves protect the soil from erosion by softening the rainfall and, especially following deforestation, by providing shade. There are about 100 species in the *Cecropia* family, *Cecropia Palmata* and *Cecropia Peltata* are the best known. The fruit it bears is a favorite food of toucans and other birds and animals. Small ants living in the hollow trunk protect the tree from other insect invaders.

Crushed leaves added to bath water were used as a relief for rheumatism.

The leaves have been known as an effective remedy that lowers blood pressure, has diuretic properties and is beneficial in cases of diabetes.

Latex resin applied externally was used to get rid of warts.

For minor fractures a poultice of fresh leaves was applied on the affected area.

For minor fractures a poultice of fresh leaves was applied on the affected area.

Decoction of leaves with a bit of honey may be used as a rinse for scorpion stings.

"The world is dialectical. Quality is influenced by quantity." Georges Ohsawa

# trees of the forest

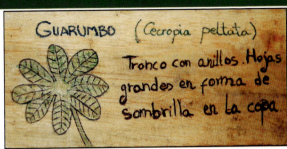

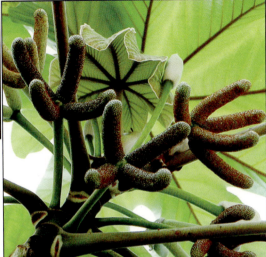

Above: A drawing of *guarumbo* used by local herbalists to pass on their knowledge about regional medicinal plants.

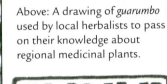

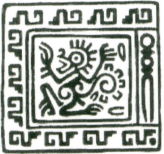

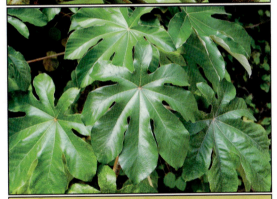

Left: The rings on the stem left from fallen leaves provide an accurate record of every petiole a particular tree ever bore. Spacing between rings indicates growing conditions during the tree's life span.

Below right: Dry leaves were sometimes smoked as bush tobacco.

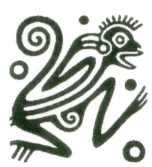

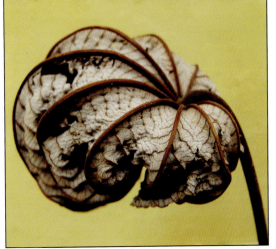

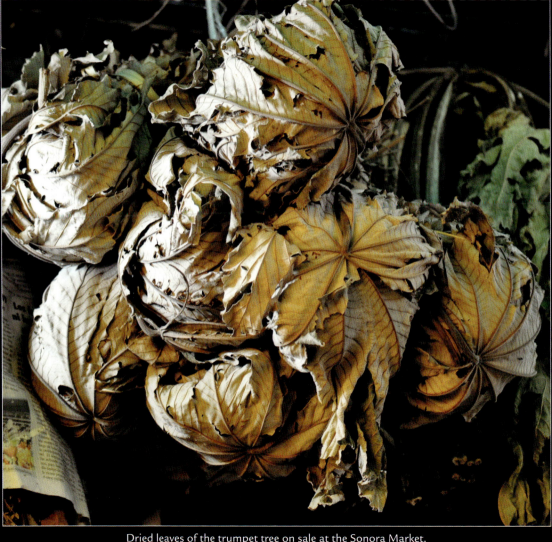
Dried leaves of the trumpet tree on sale at the Sonora Market.

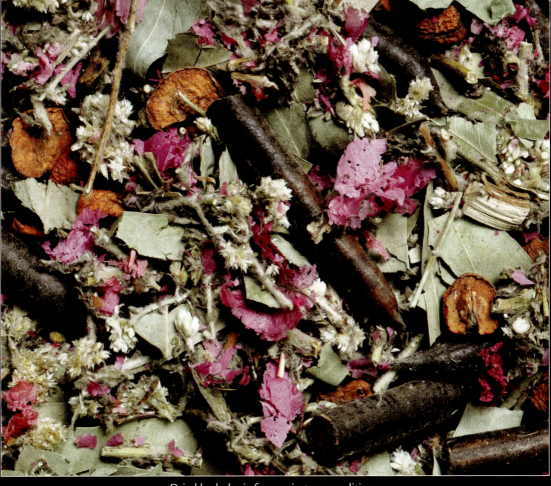
Dried herbal mix for respiratory conditions.

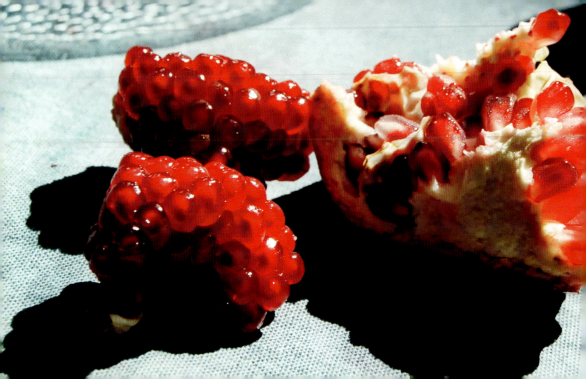

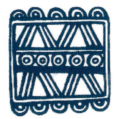
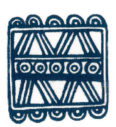
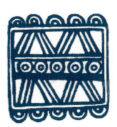
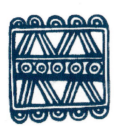
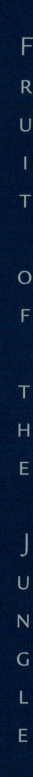

FRUIT OF THE JUNGLE

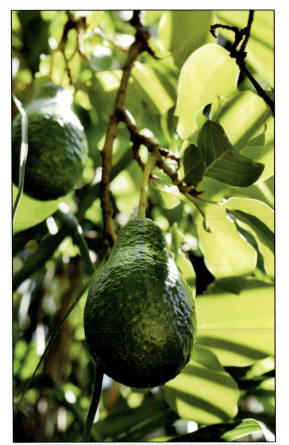

# Avocado

## Spanish Name: Aguacate
### Scientific Name: Persea americana Mill.

Avocado fruit is a very good tonic for the respiratory and nervous systems, with very beneficial properties for eyesight and circulation.

Infusion made with avocado leaves is helpful for headaches, sore throat and common colds. It may also be used to regulate the menstrual cycle.

In cases of bad digestion a few fresh leaves are boiled in 2 glasses of water and the liquid is taken warm twice a day.

A paste made with 8-10 g of avocado skin taken with water in the morning on an empty stomach gets rid of intestinal worms.

A decoction of grated seeds boiled for 10 minutes with honey is beneficial for asthma and the respiratory system.

One spoon of toasted and powdered avocado seed mixed in a glass of hot water is used as a one-time diuretic.

For high cholesterol 10 avocado leaves are mashed in 1 l of water and taken for 2 days as a drink.

A poultice made with grated avocado seeds and leaves preserved in alcohol and applied on the affected area provides quick relief for rheumatism, sprains, and pain in the joints.

Green oily fruit pulp can be applied on the face, neck and scalp as a nurturing mask.

Avocado is a beautiful tree that grows to up to 25 m in height, with alternately arranged, evergreen leaves. Avocado originated in Mexico and its characteristics vary greatly depending on the zone in which it grows. It is cultivated in Puebla, Michoacán and the entire south-east area. Guatemalan varieties are famous for the difference in size and color: from green to dark brown. An average avocado tree produces about 150 avocados annually. The avocado fruit does not ripen on the tree, it will fall off or is picked in a hard green state and later ripens quickly.

In cases of neuralgia it is recommended to rub the affected area with a dry towel in order to activate the blood circulation and then apply the liquid squeezed out of finely grated avocado seed. After that the area is covered with warm natural cloth.

Oil extracted from avocado seed is effective against hair loss, dandruff, rheumatism and gout. It may be mixed with a carrier oil and applied on affected area.

Dried and ground up avocado skin mixed with water was used as a remedy for diarrhea.

## fruit of the jungle

Avocados are extremely rich in vitamins A, E, C, K, B6, potassium, and have powerful antioxidant properties. Avocados are beautiful and delicious when used in salads, sushi, guacamole or as a complement for any Mexican plate. One medium sized fresh avocado has around 350 calories. Avocado fruits range from 200 g to more than 1 kg each. Tastes vary depending on oil content.

Guacamole is a popular Mexican dish and simple to make: mix mashed avocado, lime juice, finely chopped cilantro, onions and tomatoes with a pinch of salt.

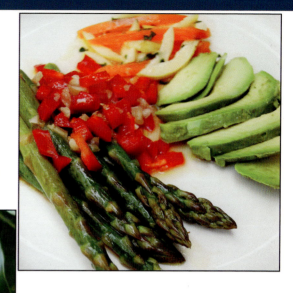

Above: Steamed asparagus served with avocado, *guayava*, red and yellow bell peppers in a citrus dressing with parsley and olive oil.

Left: Avocado flowers and small avocado fruit.

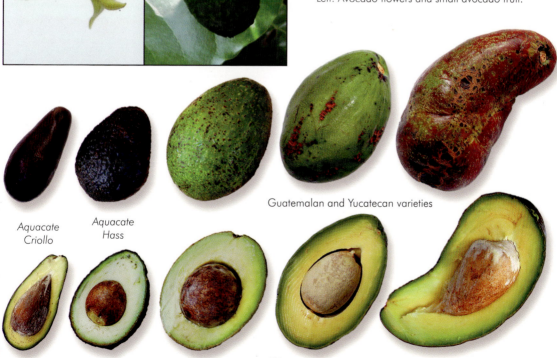

Aquacate Criollo

Aquacate Hass

Guatemalan and Yucatecan varieties

# Banana

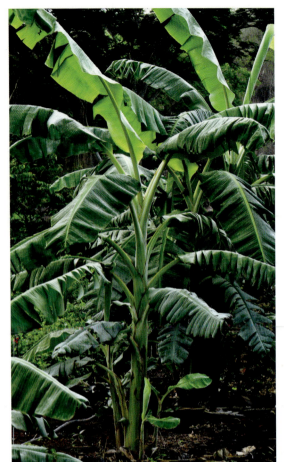

The banana is one of the most well known and liked fruits in the world. It has been used for so long that its origin is difficult to establish. It appears in some ancient records of the Incas but is also thought of being of Asian origin. Banana trees can grow rather tall and have a soft, fibrous trunk. There are many different varieties in Central and South America though nutritionally they are all very similar. Bananas have a high sugar content; from 17% to 20%.

## Spanish Name: Plátano
### Scientific Name: Musa balbisiana

Juice from the stem is rich in potassium. It was traditionally used as a remedy for tuberculosis. It is also very good for diabetes, kidney and bladder stones.

Young leaves may be applied as a relief for burns.

Bananas should only be eaten when ripe; if consumed when green they cause indigestion. Ripe bananas are very good for gastritis and diarrhea.

Because of its high protein content and alkalizing effect bananas are recommended for people with kidney and liver problems because it promotes the good function of these organs.

Banana leaves boost appetite and enhance the taste of the food which is cooked in them. The leaves are used to serve food in native cultures.

Crushed oxidized banana pulp is used to cure gastric ulcers.

Eating ripe bananas when nursing promotes milk supply.

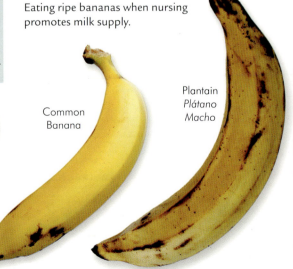

Lady Fingers
*Plátano Dominicana*

Red Cuban
*Plátano Rojo*

Common Banana

Plantain
*Plátano Macho*

# fruit of the jungle

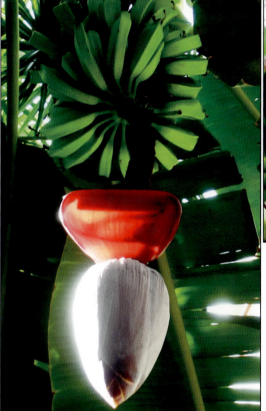

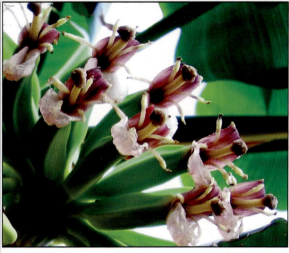

Bananas are very rich in carbohydrates, 23 g out of 100 g of fruit, so they are a very good source of energy. They are also rich in such minerals as potassium, calcium, phosphorus, sodium, iron, Vitamin C, carotene and riboflavin. Potassium helps to revitalize muscle fibers and is also a very important mineral for the proper function of the liver, calcium is necessary for bones and teeth, while phosphorus is beneficial for the nervous system.

Below left: Plantain, or *platano macho,* is not eaten raw but prepared in a variety of snacks or used as an ingredient in many dishes. When slightly unripe it is used for making banana chips.

Below right: When very ripe the plantain is baked until it breaks open, cut from one end to another, then butter, lime juice, cinnamon and honey are added while it is still hot to make a popular breakfast plate.

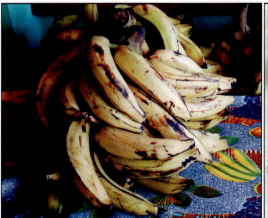

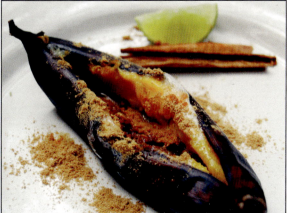

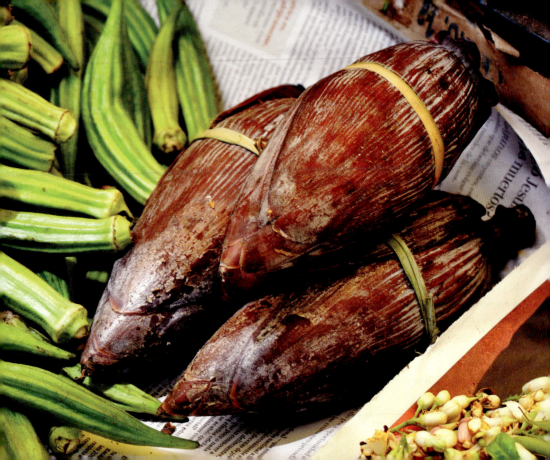

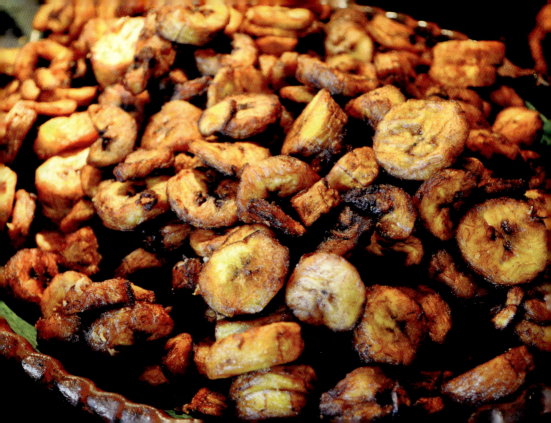

# Tamales

The *tamale* is a cornmeal pie that is made with many different ingredients. They are popular throughout Mexico and the filling depends on the regional specialties. The most popular tamales in Yucatan are usually made with corn dough, black beans and chili and tomato salsa.

To prepare *tamales* raw corn dough is rolled and placed on a banana leaf, filled with ingredients, wrapped and either steam-cooked or baked. Corn husks are another popular wrapping. Specially cured banana leaves are sold in the markets to be used for making *tamales* (below left).

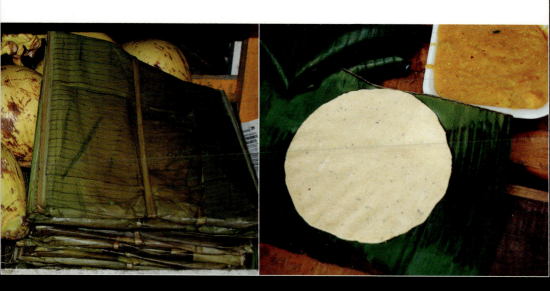

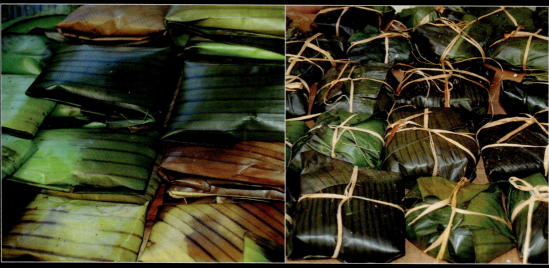

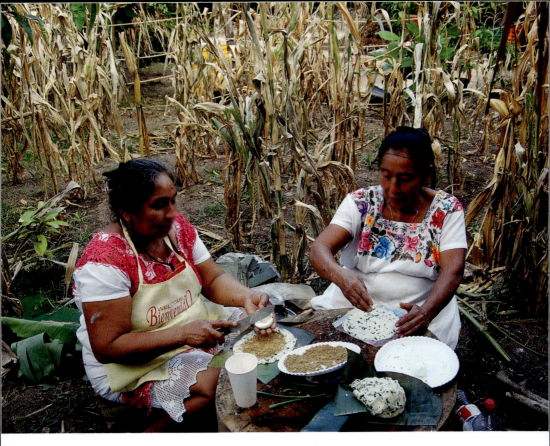

A well known Mayan specialty is *Brazo de Reina,* made for the *Janal Pixan* feast. The corn dough is mixed with chaya leaves cut in small pieces and the filling is made of ground pumpkin seeds, hardboiled egg and tomato sauce. *Brazo de Reina* is only found locally and during the festivities of *Janal Pixan*.

*Tamales* may be steamed or baked in a *pib* (left), a traditional Mayan way of preparing meals by baking them in hot coals underground. The coals are layered with palm leaves to prevent the food from burning.

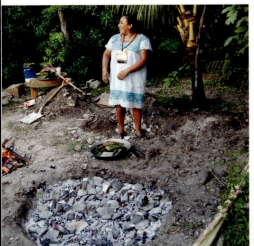
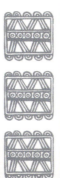
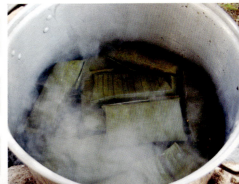

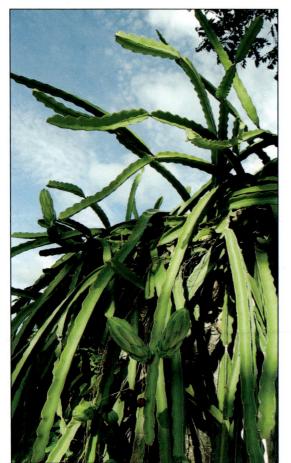

# Dragonfruit

## Spanish Name: Pitahaya
### Scientific Name: Hylocereus undatus

The flowers in an infusion are used as a heart tonic.

The fruit is diuretic and very cooling and refreshing for the body when combined with *tuna* fruit in drinks. Eating *pitahaya* lowers cholesterol levels and alleviates stomach disorders.

*Pitahaya* fruit is very beneficial for people with diabetes and minor endocrine disorders.

*Pitahaya* fruit is very rich in fiber, vitamin C and minerals. It is an antioxidant and prevents the formation of free radicals in the body.

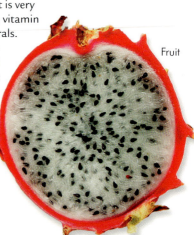

Fruit

The flowers may be eaten raw.

Dragonfruit, or strawberry pear, is the fruit of a cacti species native to Central and South America. It is widely cultivated in southeast Asia, Vietnam and China, where a yellow variety is also very common. It grows in thickets, on rocks, or on old, large tree stumps. The pitahaya flowers open at night and are called Moonflower or Queen of the Night.

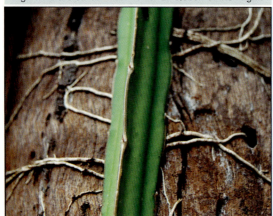

"Many times an illness begins when one is unaware of an inbalance that has subtly begun."
Huang Di, The Yellow Emperor

# fruit of the jungle

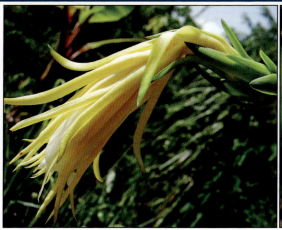
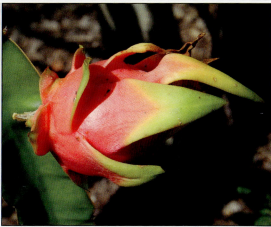

The fruit takes 30-50 days to ripen on the cactus. It can have 5-7 cycles of harvests in one year.

It is best to eat *pitahaya* cold, or it could be made into a drink. A syrup made from the whole fruit may be used to color pastries and other desserts.

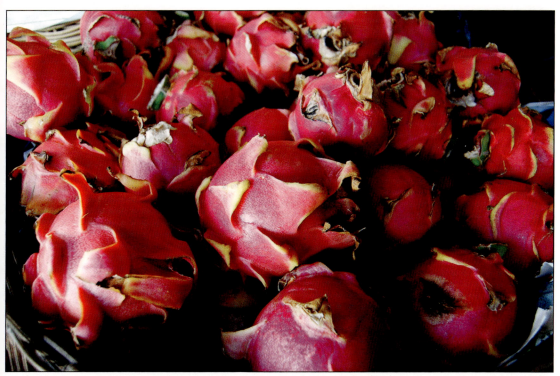

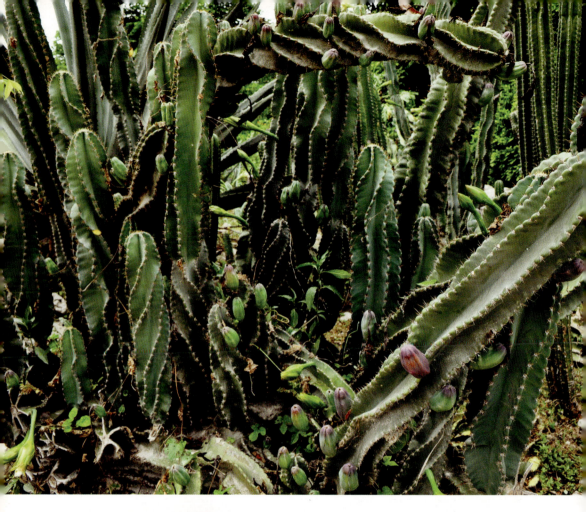

# Queen of the Night
## Selenicereus Family

There are a few dozen species in the *Selenicereus* family, all very common to the Yucatan Peninsula. A lot of them are referred to as "Queen of the Night", because their large flowers open after sunset. Most have ribbed stems and can be from 1 cm to 10 cm in diameter. The fruit of some species resemble dragonfruit and is a favorite of many birds.

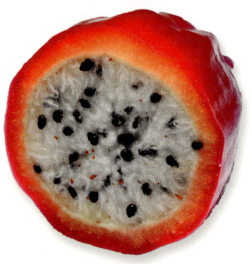

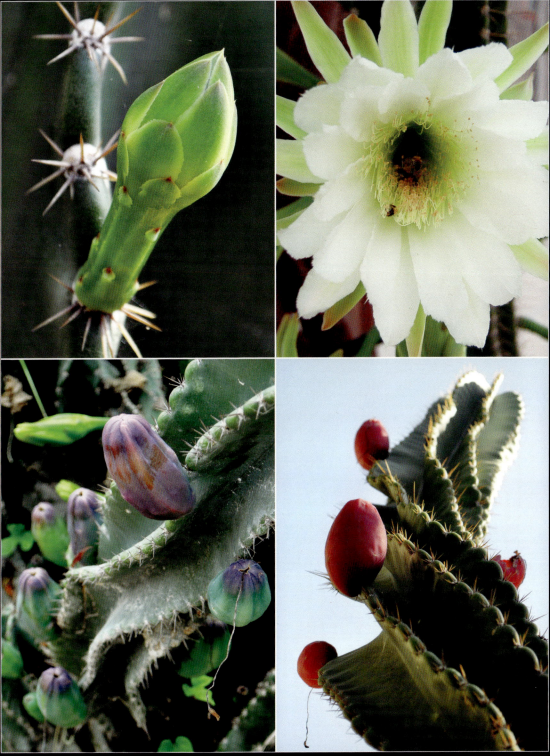

# Lime

### Spanish Name: Limón
### Scientific Name: Citrus aurantifolia

To promote sweating an infusion of chamomile and ginger is sweetened with honey, mixed with the juice of half a lime and taken while warm. After that it is recommended to stay in bed well covered.

Lime juice mixed with honey and garlic is a good expectorant; it promotes productive cough and is a good remedy for bronchitis.

Lime juice taken with warm water in the morning is excellent for the liver, kidneys and spleen and has a cleansing effect.

Lime juice is an anti-septic for minor skin infections and external irritations.

A paste made of whole limes with dark green skin was traditionally applied on snake bites.

A drop of juice in a glass of purified water may be used to disinfect the eyes.

Lime juice applied on hair brings out natural highlights and provides nutrition.

Dry lemon juice until it turns into powder and sprinkle it on books, kitchen cabinets and shelves as an insecticide.

For general cleansing effect drink mineral water with lime juice and honey added to it.

Rubbing lime on insect bites provides temporary relief.

Lime contains magnesium which is excellent for the nervous and circulatory systems.

The lime is a citrus tree usually between 3-6 m in height which thrives even in poor and rocky soil. It is from the same family as orange, bitter orange, lemon, grape fruit and citron. Lime is bright green, smaller than the lemon, more acidic, and has a thinner rind. There are several varieties that are very common in the Yucatan Peninsula, among them is *limón lima* with a most exquisite fragrance, and sweet lime, or *limón dulce*, a heirloom variety sometimes found in small farmer's markets.

"He, who eats, exists. Like all other beings man is transformation of foods."
Georges Ohsawa

# fruit of the jungle

Lime is a good condiment that adds taste, flavor and promotes digestion. High vitamin C content helps the body to better utilize other vitamins and minerals.

Lime is a popular addition to many international recipes, marinades, cocktails and desserts.

Fresh lime juice in salad dressing is a substitute for vinegar; make any flavor by adding your favorite ingredient: mustard, raspberries, garlic, herbs, sesame seeds, dry cheese, olive oil, sea salt and a few drops of honey.

Despite its sour taste, lime has an alkalizing effect on the body.

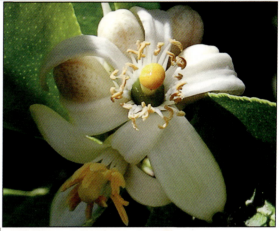

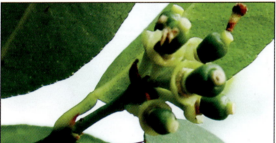

Instead of using commercial food disinfectants it is recommended to soak vegetables or clean fruit in a strong lime juice and water solution.

Lime extracts and essential oils are frequently used in aromatherapy and natural household products.

Essence of lemon is anti-bacterial, anti-viral, is a good digestive tonic and may be used externally mixed in equal amounts with carrier oil for acne, warts and herpes. A couple of drops of lemon essential oil taken with a spoon of honey daily is believed to facilitate the work of internal organs, resulting in gradual detoxification. **Not recommended during pregnancy.**

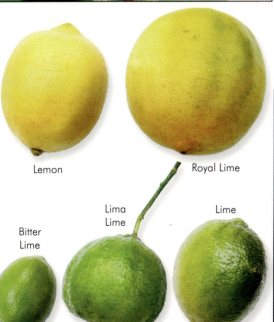

Lemon    Royal Lime

Lima Lime    Lime

Bitter Lime

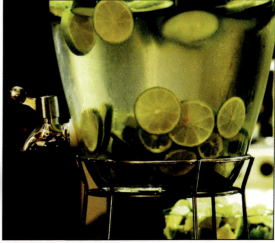

# Mango

## Spanish Name: Mango
### Scientific Name: Mangifera indica L.

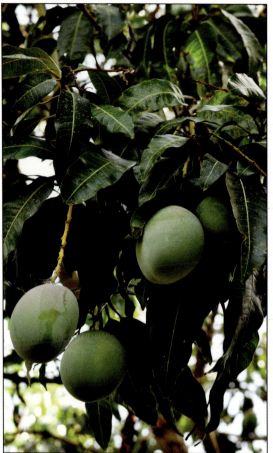

The Mango tree is one of the most significant trees on the planet, and one of the oldest cultivated trees. It is native to Southern Asia: Burma or India. Mangos are referred to as the "food of the gods" in the Hindu Vedas. Mango trees can live for centuries, with some over 300 years old and still producing fruit. The trees are large, reaching 35-40 m in height, with a crown radius of 10 m. The leaves are evergreen and the fruit takes from three to six months to ripen. Mango fruit has the best flavor if it is allowed to ripen on the tree. All parts of the mango tree are used in traditional medicine: fruit, seeds, flowers, leaves, bark and even resin that comes out of the trunk.

Mango leaves and bark are believed to inhibit the growth of bacteria.

Infusion of leaves is astringent and is a remedy for cough and asthma.

Dried flowers were used as a cure for dysentery.

Bark has a very beneficial effect on the mucous membrane and a decoction is taken for chronic diarrhea.

Dry skin of the fruit is an expectorant when taken in an infusion.

Ripe mango fruit is very good for the heart muscle, liver, kidneys and it stimulates the appetite. Eating mango is beneficial for people who suffer from frequent headaches.

In tropical parts of Mexico raw or ripe mango served with chile and salt is an excellent thirst quencher that prevents the body from losing sodium and iron during the summer months as a result of excessive sweating.

Eating a lot of mangoes when they are in season supports the formation of healthy skin tissues, epithelium, due to a very high content of Vitamin A.

Chewing mango leaves is a remedy for bleeding gums.

Green unripe mangoes have very high content of Vitamin C; eating them in moderation increases the elasticity of the blood vessels and promotes the formation of new blood cells. The acid in green mangoes stimulates the secretion of bile and acts as a general gastrointestinal antiseptic.

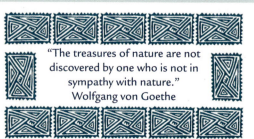

"The treasures of nature are not discovered by one who is not in sympathy with nature."
Wolfgang von Goethe

# fruit of the jungle

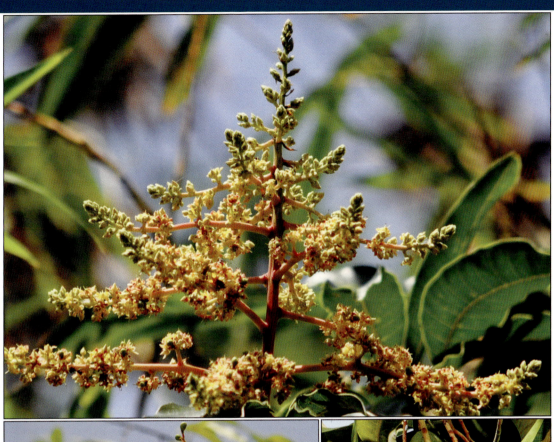
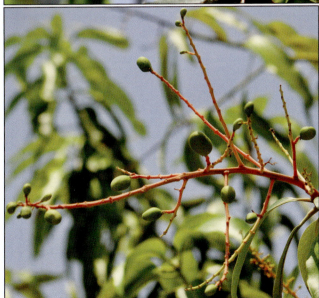
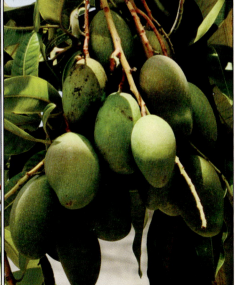

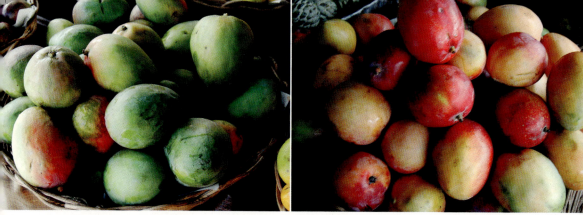

## Enjoy mango season from February to August!

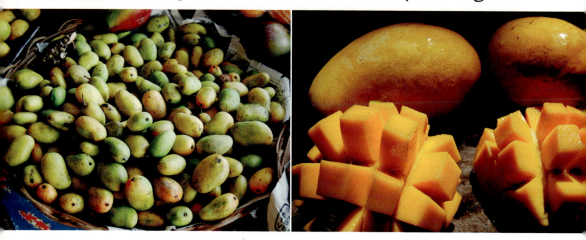

Mangoes are everybody's favorite and are widely used in chutneys, sauces, desserts, sherbets and ice cream. Fresh juice is delicious and so are liquados in combination with papaya, pineapple, orange or kiwi! In Mexico green unripe mangoes are used to make salsa with chile, lime and cilantro. In India mango leaves are used in prayers to please the gods and are known as the paisley design in textiles.

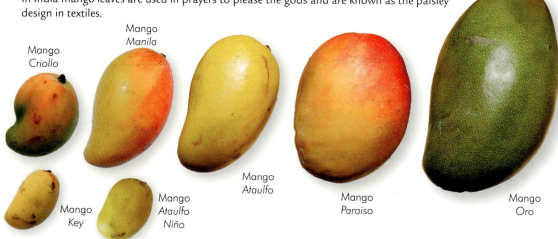

Mango Criollo · Mango Manila · Mango Ataulfo · Mango Paraiso · Mango Oro · Mango Key · Mango Ataulfo Niño

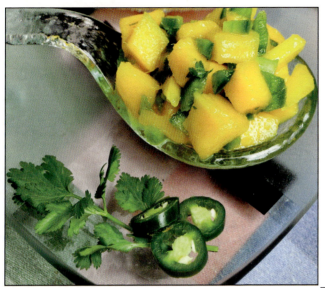

# Mango salsas

Even in Mexico, a country with a dozen varieties of mangoes, this fruit is only available when it is in season. It starts in the end of February and can last until fall. Mango salsa is a gourmet condiment which is becoming more and more popular. Fresh salsa is best when served chilled. Slightly cooked warm mango salsa can be made into a chutney or salad dressing.

The ingredients are finely chopped, combined and set to cool for about 20 minutes before serving. They may accompany chips, crackers, cheese, dinner plates or appetizers.

## Ripe mango salsa

Mango *ataulfo* or *paraíso*
Chile *árbol/Serrano/jalapeño*
Cilantro or mint
Lime juice
A pinch of salt

## Warm mango salsa

Mangoes are mashed or blended and cloves, cinnamon, lime or orange juice, nuts and raisins are added while the mix is cooked for about 5 minutes. This warm sauce may be added to dishes, salads, baked desserts, crepes, cheese plates and ice creams or sorbet. If refrigerated it may be served with custard or flan.

Below: Ripe *guayava* halves filled with fresh mango salsa.

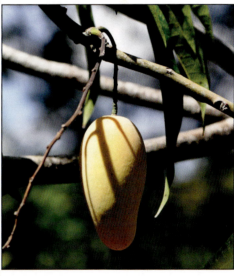

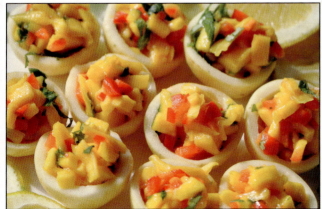

## Green mango salsa

Unripe mango oro or criollo
Chile habañero
Salt and lime juice
Cilantro or mint

# Nopal

## Spanish Name: Nopal
### Scientific Name: Opuntia ficus-indica L.

Nopal is a large cactus native to Mexico which may be as tall as 4-5 m with many waxy pads covered with spikes. Bright colorful flowers bloom along the edges and attract local stingless bees. It is very common throughout the Yucatan, growing wild and cultivated in gardens of small towns and sold at the markets cleaned of spikes and ready to use. *Tuna* is the fruit of nopal, it may vary in color from pale green to bright purple when ripe.

Flowers, pads and fruit are valued for their medicinal or nutritional properties. Fresh juice from one pad mixed with water is recommended as a preventative remedy excellent for diabetes, weak lungs, inflammation of the spleen and during difficult childbirth.

A remedy for headache and fever is made of one sliced nopal pad boiled with 3 cups of water for 5 minutes. 1 cup of strained liquid is taken before each meal during one day. This same remedy is believed to be helpful in cases of mild hypertension, bladder problems and for hair loss prevention.

Using nopal in the diet is very good for people with arthritis.

For minor skin rashes and burns pads are split open and the internal side is applied directly to the skin.

A solution made out of nopal flowers has an astringent action: it shrinks and tightens the top layer of the skin reducing lines and improving tissue firmness.

**NOT RECOMMENDED during pregnancy and while breast feeding.**

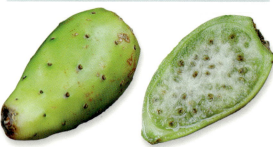

The *tuna* fruits are eaten raw or made into jelly. The juice extracted from pads or fruits is a healthy drink.

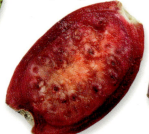
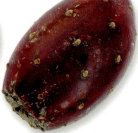

# fruit of the jungle

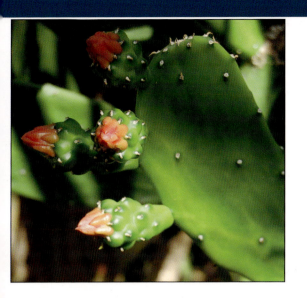

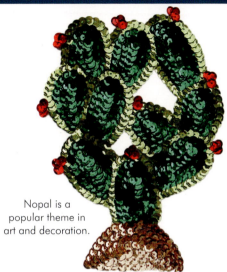

Nopal is a popular theme in art and decoration.

## Try nopal salad - it's healty and delicious!

After the spikes are removed almost the entire plant may be used for food. Pads from young plants are sliced and cooked as a vegetable. They have a light, slightly tart flavor and a crisp, mucilaginous texture.

Nopal is very rich in insoluble and soluble dietary fibers, vitamins A, C, K, riboflavin, B6 and such minerals as magnesium, potassium, manganese, iron and copper.

Try it in salads! Nopales are widely used in Mexican cuisine: huevos con nopales, eggs with nopal, or tacos de nopales are among the most favorite.

The entire pad may be marinated, grilled, and served as a side dish or as an appetizer.

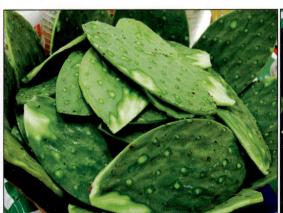

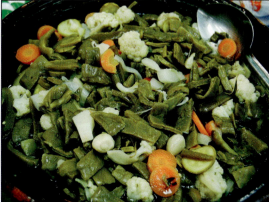

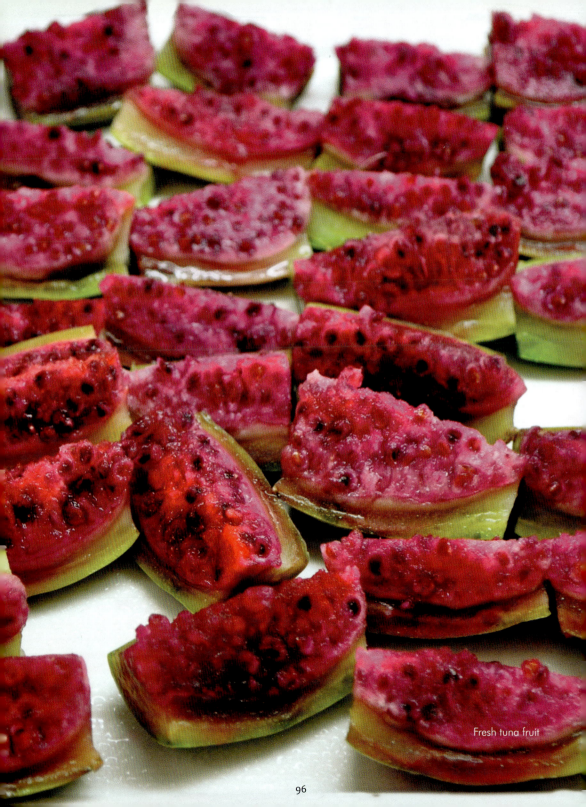

Fresh tuna fruit

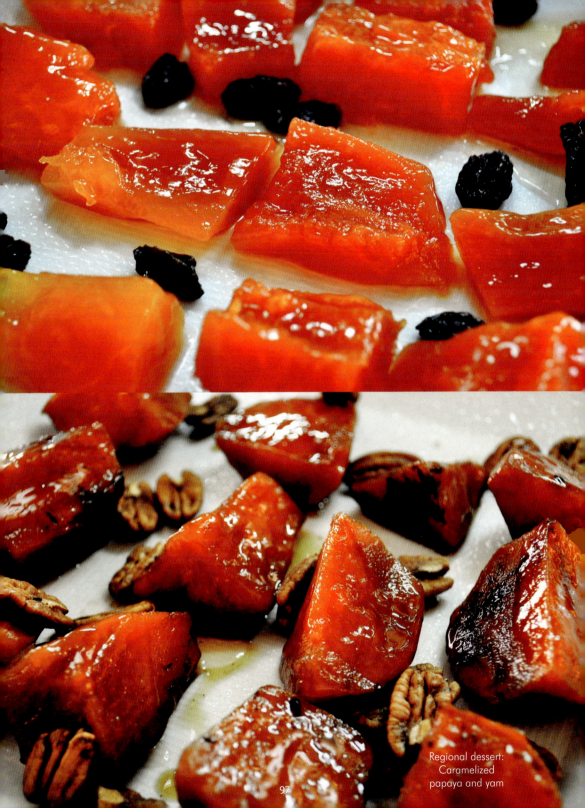

Regional dessert: Caramelized papaya and yam

# Papaya

**SPANISH NAME: PAPAYA**
**SCIENTIFIC NAME: CARICA PAPAYA L.**

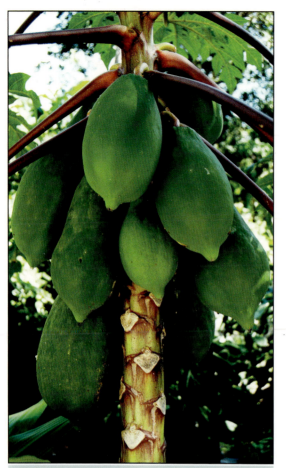

Papaya is native to tropical America. It is a large plant that reaches from 3-10 m. It likes dry soil and a lot of sun. If it is irrigated exsessively the roots may start rotting. When the fruit is green and hard it is rich in white latex. Ripe papaya is juicy, sweet and has a unique flavor. Attached lightly to the inner wall are hundreds of small black seeds. From healthy plants from 40 kg to 150 kg of fruit per year may be harvested. There are several types of papaya in Mexico; the most common in the Yucatan Peninsula is the large red and yellow variety often called papaya maradol.

Dr. Hulda Clark recommends papaya leaves as an anti-cancer remedy with the following recipe: wash and cut into pieces several medium sized papaya leaves, then cook in 2 l of water until the water reduces in half. 3 tbsp. are taken 3 times a day.

10 papaya seeds are taken daily on an empty stomach for one week against intestinal parasites. The seeds may be swallowed whole or chewed.

The fruit as well as other parts of the plant are rich in papain, an enzyme that helps to digest proteins

An infusion made with flowers or very young leaves is beneficial for cough and asthma.

The white resin from green fruit diluted with water in proportion 1:10 (1 part resin, 10 parts water) and a few drops of honey is considered a good remedy for arthritis, tuberculosis and high blood pressure.

In folk medicine the fresh white resin from green fruit is used to get rid of warts.

Slices of fruit applied on skin irritations and fire coral burns are believed to alleviate discomfort.

Young leaves may be steamed and eaten like spinach.

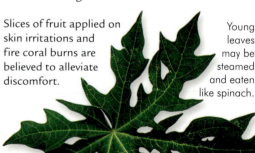

Papaya is a good source of iron, calcium and vitamins A, B, and C.

# fruit of the jungle

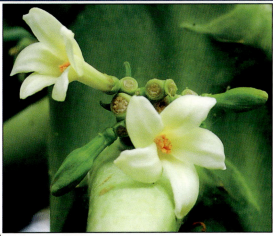

Papaya seeds contain over 18 amino acids. They are edible and are sometimes ground up and used as a substitute for black pepper.

It is a popular fruit to enjoy with any type of breakfast. A popular snack in Mexico is papaya sprinkled with red chile and lime juice. Papaya is also used in salads, sorbets, juices and dried with other fruits in granola. Green unripe fruit can be cooked like squash.

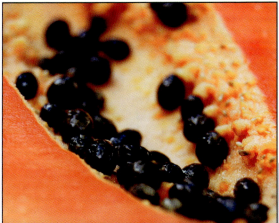

Papayas have light yellow, waxy and pleasantly fragrant female flowers very close to the stem. At the same time papayas give small male flowers that are clustered on a long shoot. It is possible for the same plant to have both male and female flowers. Fresh female flowers have a very pleasant fragrance and are a good addition to any herbal infusion.

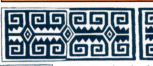
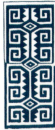

"To Goethe the fact that the action of the root of a plant is directed earthward towards moisture and darkness, whereas stem or trunk strives skyward in the opposite direction toward the light and the air, was a truly magical phenomenon."
The Secret Life of Plants

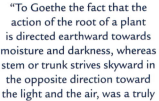
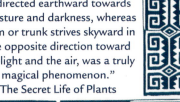
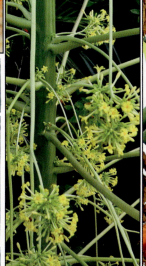
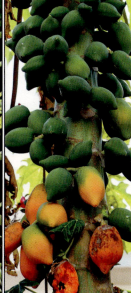
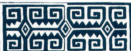

# Pomegranate

### SPANISH NAME: GRANADA
### SCIENTIFIC NAME: PUNICA GRANATUM L.

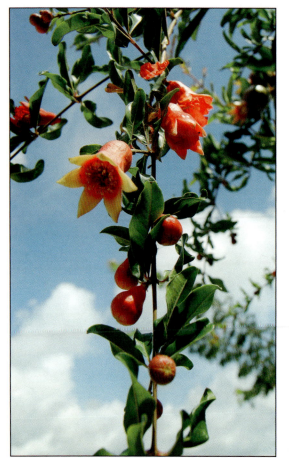

The pomegranate is a tree that grows up to 6-7 m in height and has a life span up to 200 years. It is believed to be native to the Himalayas, but since ancient times it has been cultivated in the Mediterranean region, India, and Southeast Asia. It was introduced to Central America, and the variety common to Mexico has a smaller fruit. Pomegranates are famous for their beautiful scarlet red or white flowers.

Pomegranate has astringent qualities and fresh juice is a tonic and purifier for the entire body.

The entire seed of the pomegranate may be eaten raw or just the juice squeezed out. The taste can be from very sweet to sour and tangy.

A delicious thick sauce can be made with pomegranate juice and walnuts.

Pomegranate molasses is pomegranate syrup further reduced and is a delicious product that may be used for sauces, salad dressings and desserts.

Dried skin and internal fiber in infusion is a great remedy against diarrhea and is safe for children and adults.
The entire dried and fire roasted fruit ground into powder and taken as infusion is another local remedy for diarrhea.

Pomegranate has been used as a skin tonic. A light, wet massage of face and neck with pomegranate juice improves circulation, color, and has a rejuvenating effect.

Leaves in bath are an effective cure for minor skin eruptions, pimples, skin parasites or itching.

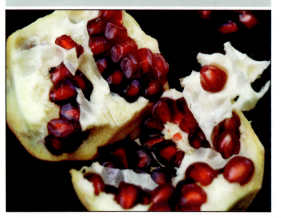

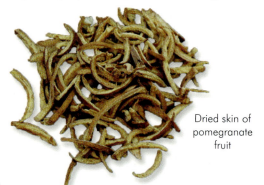

Dried skin of pomegranate fruit

# fruit of the jungle

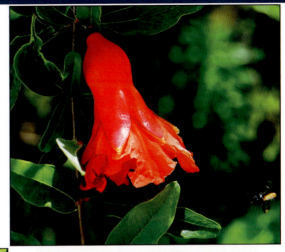

If the branches are trimmed during the 14 days following the full moon the plant will flower and produce fruit much faster. If you trim them again after the fruit is harvested it will flower in a short time.

Pomegranate fruit is rich in mineral salts such as potassium, phosphorus, sodium, magnesium, calcium, and it has good quantities of Vitamins C, A, and B. Delicious juices, sauces and chutneys are popular in gourmet cuisines of many cultures. The small red seeds may be used to decorate dishes, sorbets and desserts.

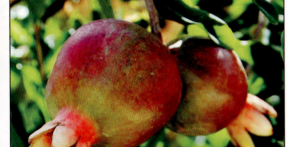

"Flowers that remain unfertilized emit a strong fragrance for as long as 8 days or until the flower withers and falls. Once impregnated the flower ceases to exude its fragrance in less than half an hour."
The Secret Life of Plants

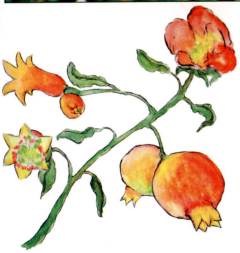

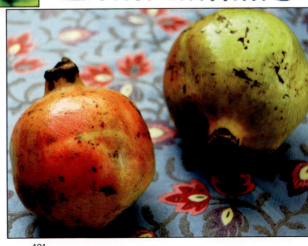

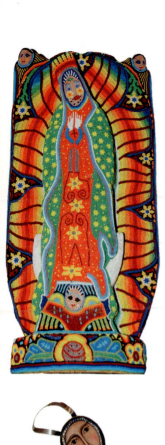
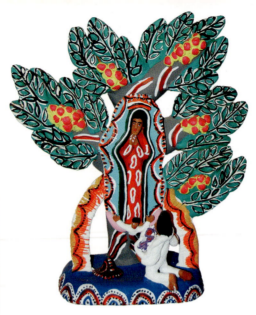
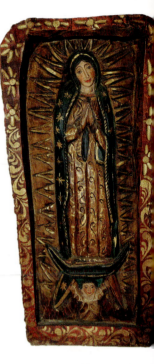
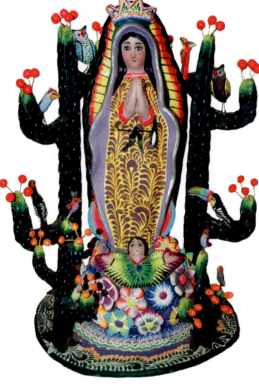
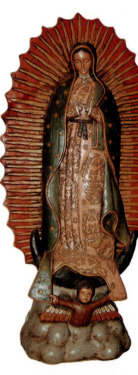

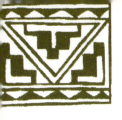
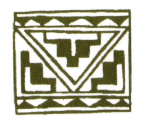
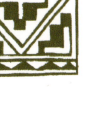

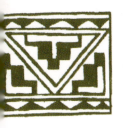

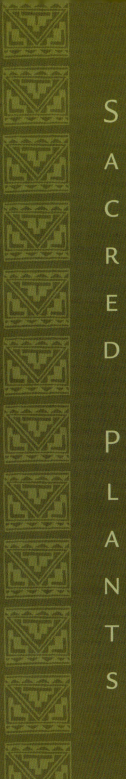

SACRED PLANTS

# Copal Tree

## Spanish Name: Copal
### Scientific Name: Bursera bipinnata

The copal tree resin is called *pom* in Mayan and is indispensable in all rituals, ceremonies and healing practices because it is believed to protect against witchcraft, ill will, bad luck and evil eye. In order to produce the fragrant smoke copal is usually sprinkled on hot coals.

Carvings and offerings of copal were excavated from the famous Chichen Itza cenote.

The berries from the copal tree were used as a cure for acne.

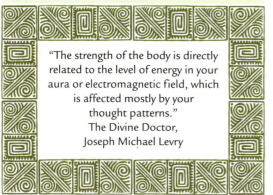

Most copal incense in Central America comes from the trees of the *Burseraceae* family, rapid growing trees able to adapt to almost any soil. They are not so common in Yucatan and most white copal sold locally comes from Oaxaca.

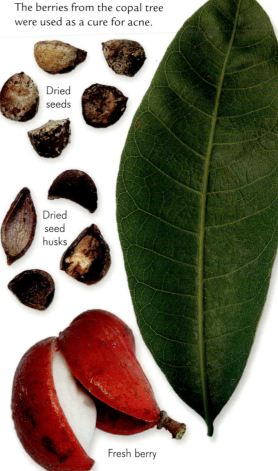

Dried seeds

Dried seed husks

Fresh berry

"The strength of the body is directly related to the level of energy in your aura or electromagnetic field, which is affected mostly by your thought patterns."
The Divine Doctor,
Joseph Michael Levry

sacred plants

# White Copal

Copal is extracted by making a deep cut in the bark and letting the resin drip out. After it dries it is scraped off. A practice of "sweating" the tree, setting a circle of fire around its trunk and thus forcing the resin to run, was used with some varieties of trees.

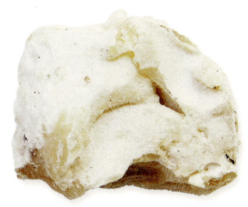

White resin from this particular tree, referred to as *pom* in Mayan, is the true copal incense.

Resin from the trees of the same family is often sold as copal. It varies in color and the amount of smoke that it produces. Each has its own distinct fragrance and may be used the same way as white copal; sprinkled on hot coals.

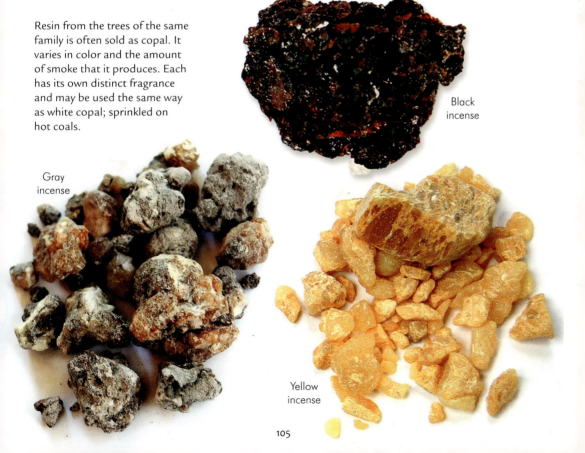

Black incense

Gray incense

Yellow incense

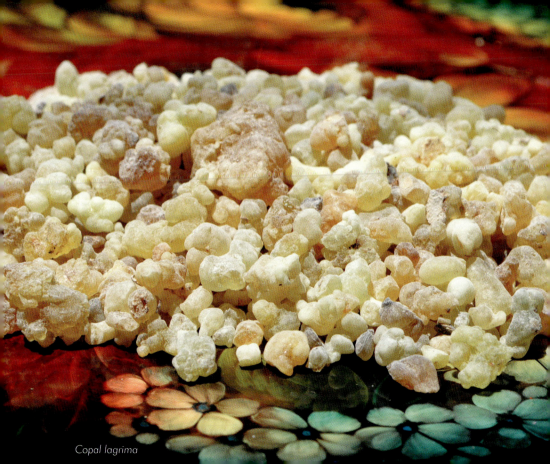
*Copal lagrima*

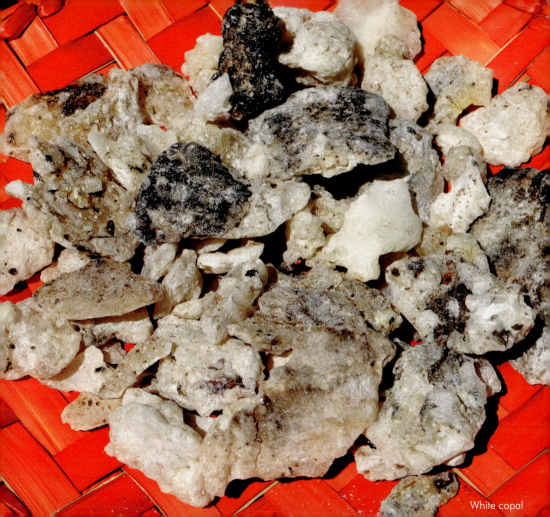

White copal

# Alebrijes

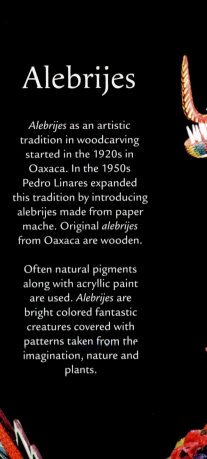

*Alebrijes* as an artistic tradition in woodcarving started in the 1920s in Oaxaca. In the 1950s Pedro Linares expanded this tradition by introducing alebrijes made from paper mache. Original *alebrijes* from Oaxaca are wooden.

Often natural pigments along with acryllic paint are used. *Alebrijes* are bright colored fantastic creatures covered with patterns taken from the imagination, nature and plants.

Copal wood is very soft when green and is the best material for the carving of *alebrijes*. They are carved while the wood is still green and placed in the sun to dry and then painted.

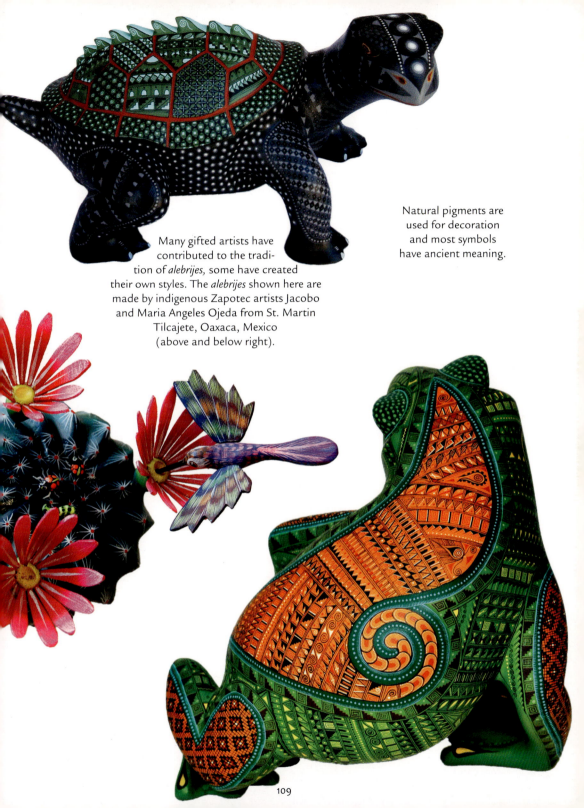

Many gifted artists have contributed to the tradition of *alebrijes*, some have created their own styles. The *alebrijes* shown here are made by indigenous Zapotec artists Jacobo and Maria Angeles Ojeda from St. Martin Tilcajete, Oaxaca, Mexico (above and below right).

Natural pigments are used for decoration and most symbols have ancient meaning.

# Corn

## Spanish Name: Maíz
### Scientific Name: Zea mays L.

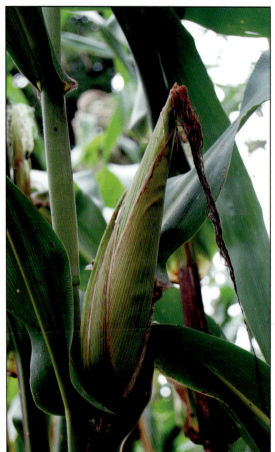

Corn silk in infusion is a well known diuretic and a good remedy for different kidney disorders and is also a bladder tonic. A cloth soaked in this infusion may be applied directly to the affected area in cases of nefritis, gout and sciatica.

Toasted corn mixed with water has astringent qualities and is a good remedy for diarrhea.

In cases of general weakness, a drink called *atole* is taken frequently with a little corn silk added to it.

In cases of hysteria, *atole* is also helpful with a few leaves of *ruda* added to it when the *atole* has been taken off the fire already.

In traditional medicine freshly made corn dough was used for bruises, ulcers, wounds, and irritations as a poultice.

Corn is indiginous to the western hemisphere and has been cultivared for thousands of years. There are four main varietes: white, yellow, blue and red. Corn grows easily and can be planted together with beans. All parts of the plant were used after harvesting. The tassle of the corn consists of many small male flowers, while the ear consists of female flowers. Each kernel is connected to a single strand of silk which all go to a point outside the ear. Corn is believed to have evolved from some of the wild grasses in the Central or South America. Corn is at present time one of the 12 most important crop plants in the world. Corn has a high starch and oil content.

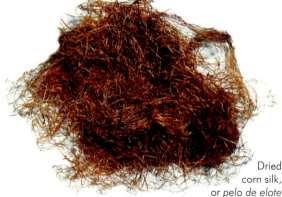

Dried corn silk, or *pelo de elote*

White corn, common in the Yucatan Peninsula.

# sacred plants

According to the *Popol Vuh,* the ancestors of the *Quiche* Maya were created from corn.

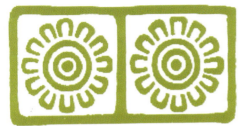

Above: Ancient Mayan stamp depicting corn.

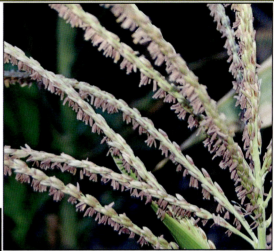

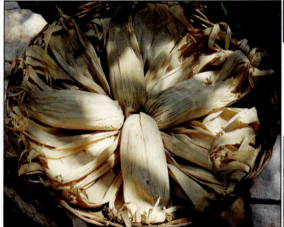

Of the four sacred plants: corn, squash, beans and tobacco – corn, of course, is the most important. No ritual can be held without corn.

Below: Traditional bag made from wool spun and woven by hand, embrioded with corn designs.

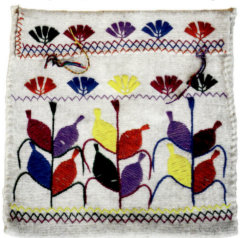

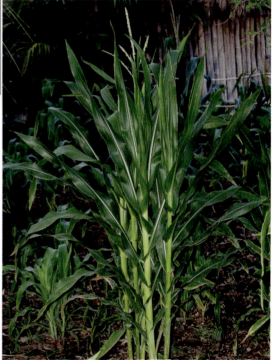

# sacred plants

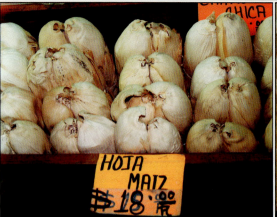
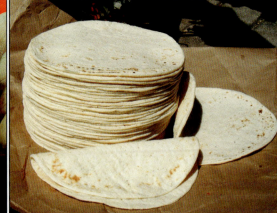

Corn is a part of almost every meal in the Yucatan. Besides *tortillas, panuchos, sopes, polkanos, flautas, chilendrines* and other variations of corn cakes there is also *pozole, tamale* and *atole,* an ancient corn drink that can be sweetend with honey and spiced with chile.

*Atole* was a part of the traditional Mayan morning meal and could be carried to the fields in a gourd. It was served hot or cold.

Fresh corn kernels mixed with finely chopped chile, cilantro, tomatillos, a pinch of salt and lime juice make a light and nutritious salsa.

For dessert on a hot day try corn ice cream, one of the unique Mexican specialties.

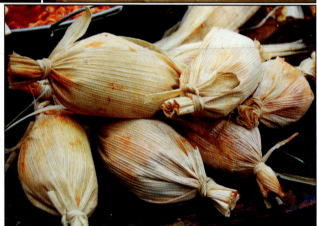

*Tamales* (above) are delicious and extremely popular in Mexico. They are made with with a variety of fillings such as beans, chaya, eggs, ground pumpkin seed, potatoes, cheese and herbs.

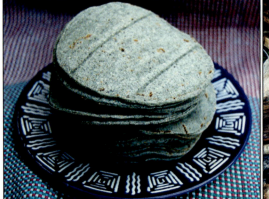
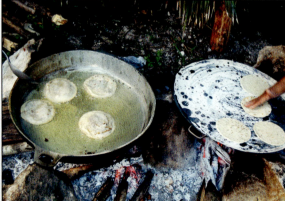

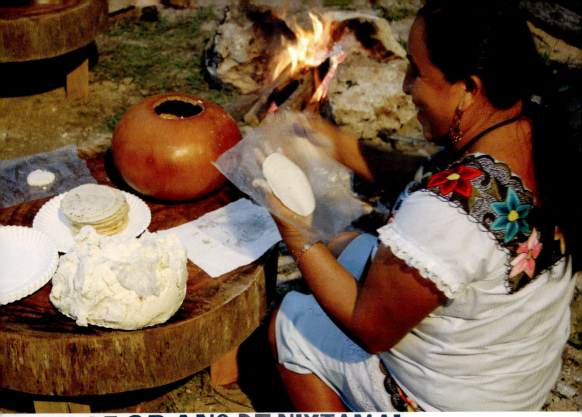

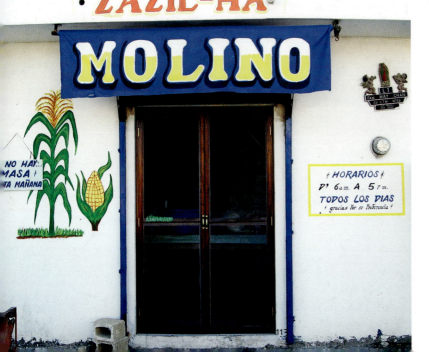

## Nixtamal

*Nixtamal* is corn dough prepared in a traditional way. The process of making *nixtamal* is believed to be about 3000 years old. Slaked lime was added to water and put to boil; when ready, previously washed corn was added. After boiling for a short time it was taken off the fire, covered and left to stand until the next day, when it was washed and ground with a mortar.

# Corn & Art

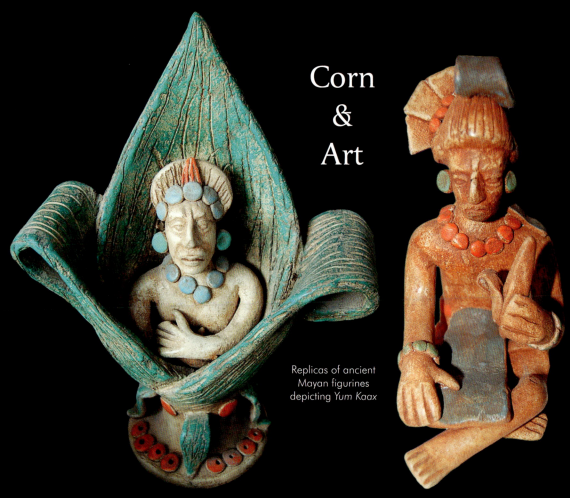

Replicas of ancient Mayan figurines depicting *Yum Kaax*

Above: Modern artists make replicas of ancient mayan sculptures using traditional dyes and materials.
Below: In *Huichol* art corn is one of the most frequently represented plants. These intricate pictures are made with colorful yarn without previous draft or design. A special wax holds the tightly placed yarn for many years.

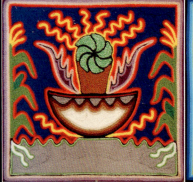
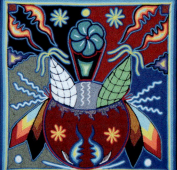
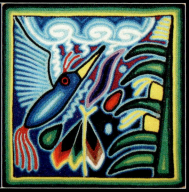

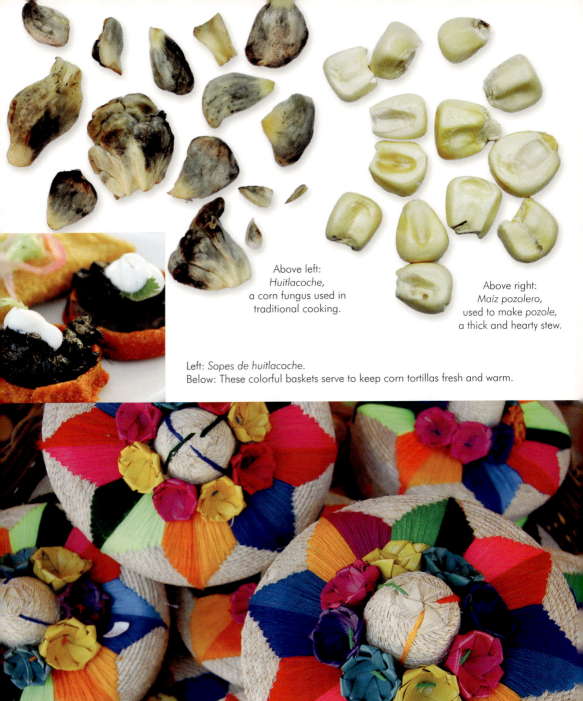

Above left:
*Huitlacoche*, a corn fungus used in traditional cooking.

Above right:
*Maíz pozolero*, used to make *pozole*, a thick and hearty stew.

Left: *Sopes de huitlacoche*.
Below: These colorful baskets serve to keep corn tortillas fresh and warm.

# Yum Kaax

*Yum Kaax* means the master of the forest. *Yum Kaax* was depicted by the ancient Maya as a youthful deity holding ears of corn in both hands. As a son of *Itzamna* and *Ixchel*, *Yum Kaax* represented a perfect intelligence that governed all the natural elements. *Yum Kaax* was associated with life, prosperity, abundance and agriculture.

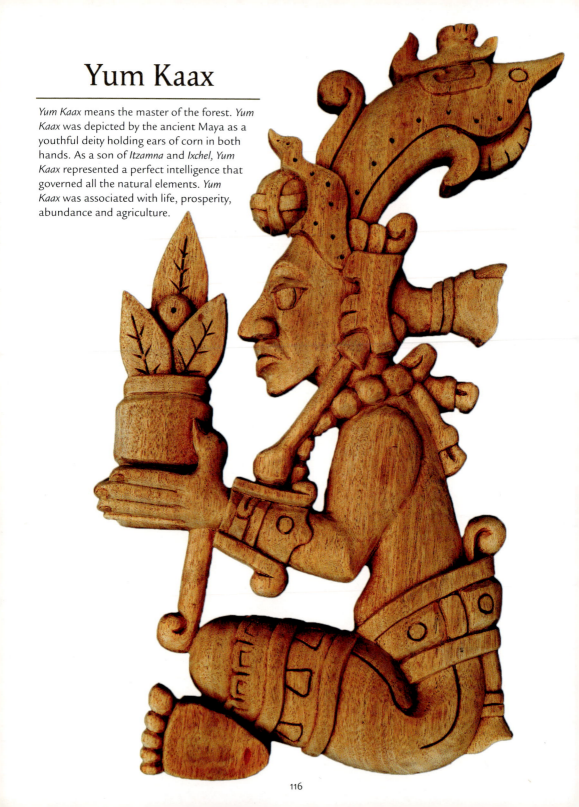

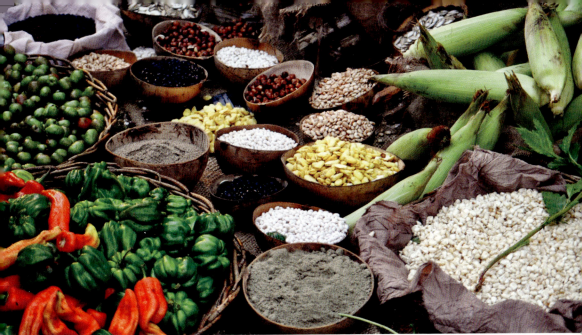

*Milpa* is a the Mesoamerican system of growing crops with the cycle based on two years of cultivation and 8 years of letting the soil recover. This system allows for large yields of food crops including corn, beans, squash, avocados, tomatoes, chiles, sweet potatoes, jicama, amaranth and *yuca*.

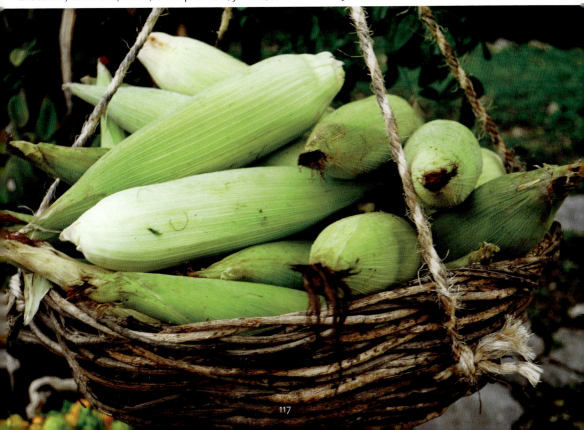

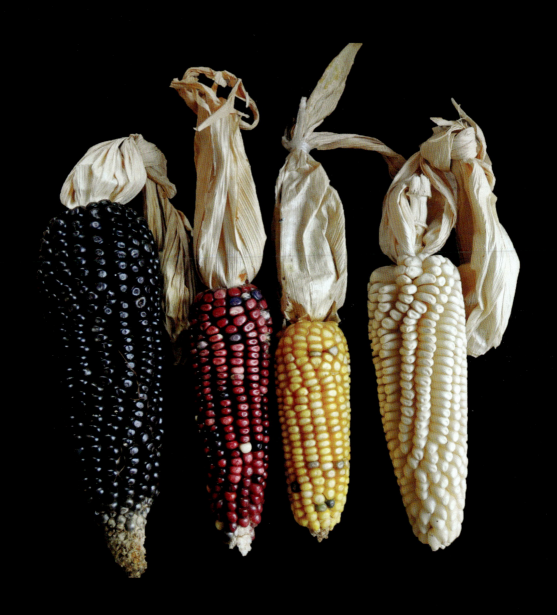

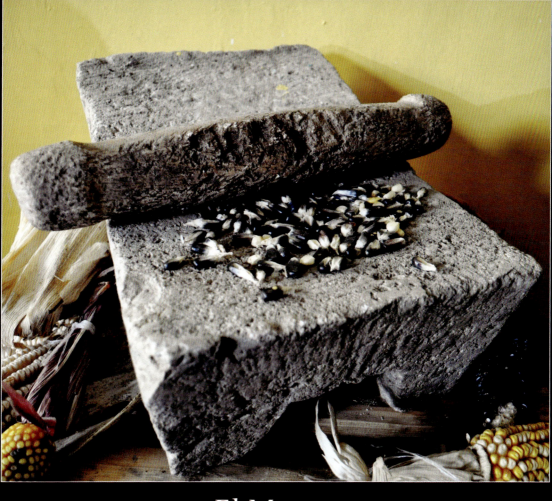

# El Metate

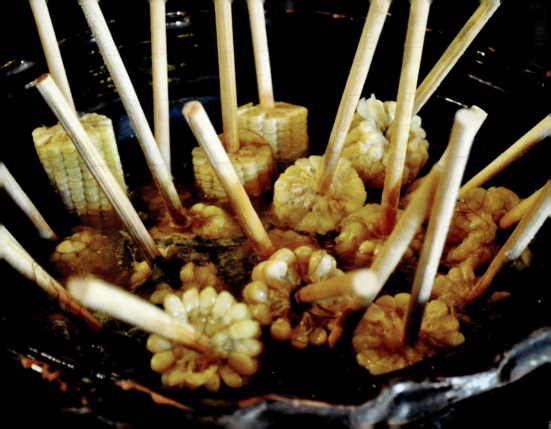

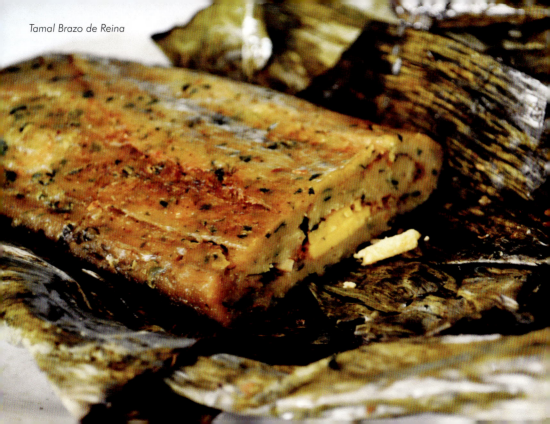
*Tamal Brazo de Reina*

**Spanish Name: Ceiba**
Scientific Name: Ceiba pentandra gaerm

# Kapok Tree

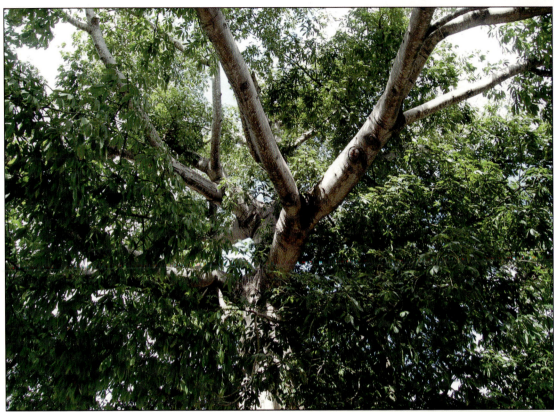

The kapok tree, or *yaxche* in Mayan, is common throughout the American tropics as well as West Africa. For the Maya, *yaxche* was a tree of life and a sacred tree. It was beleived to connect the terrestrial world with the spirit world above. The ceiba flowers were worn by kings and ceiba motifs are found in traditional textiles. Ceiba trees are among the tallest in the tropical forest, reaching a height of 70 m. The trunk was used to make dugout canoes, which are still made and used today. Ceiba fruits are pear shaped and green, up to 20 cm long, with 5 sections that split open to reveal abundant fluff, or kapok, to which small dark brown seeds are attached. Some ceiba trees flower once in 5 years.

The seeds, leaves, bark and resin all were used in traditional medicine for a wide variety of conditions including dysentery, respiratory problems and kidney disorders.

A decoction made of the boiled bark was used for inflammation, as a diuretic and an antispasmodic.

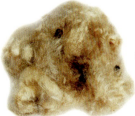 

Fluff and seeds

Ceiba seeds have a high oil and protein content and are edible. The oil was used for making soap.

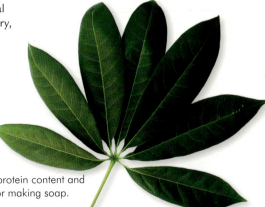

# sacred plants

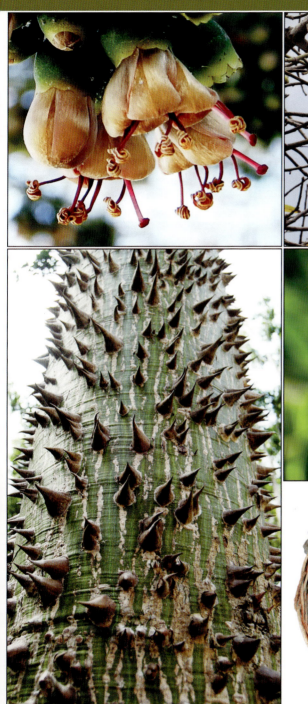
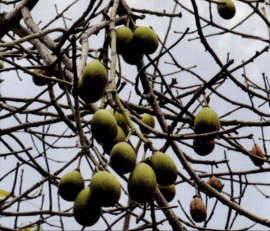
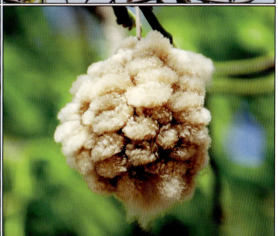
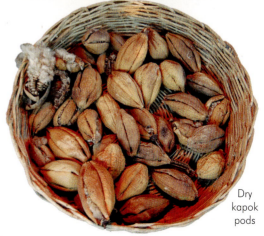

Dry kapok pods

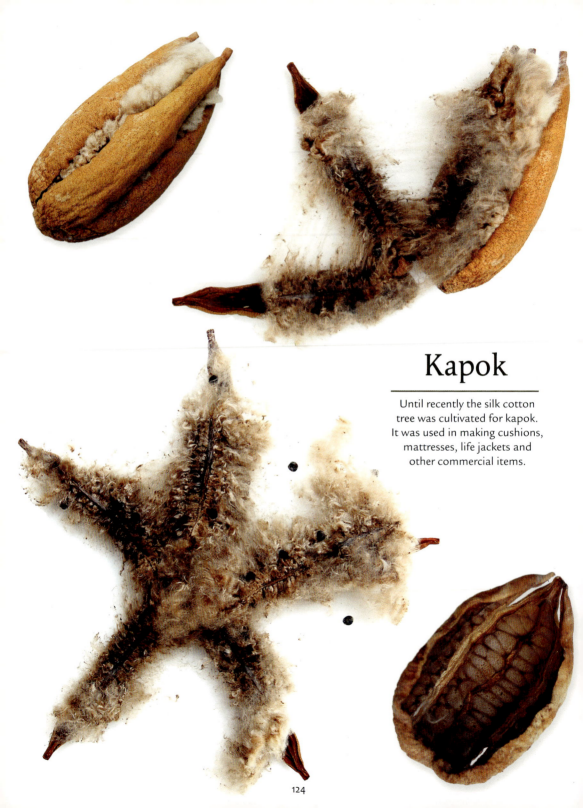

# Kapok

Until recently the silk cotton tree was cultivated for kapok. It was used in making cushions, mattresses, life jackets and other commercial items.

# Tree of Life
# Arbol de Vida

The ceiba tree loses all its leaves right before flowering. The tree stays without the leaves until the pods mature and open and the wind carries off the kapok with the seeds attached to it. As soon as all the seeds are gone new leaves appear and the life cycle begins again.

According to the Mayan myths there were four ceiba trees sustaining the sky. The myth also said that when the forest disappears the roof of the sky will crumble down.
Ceiba has a very special meaning in present day culture. It is common to receive a blessing or have a ceremony made near a ceiba tree.

The Castillo family (above right, below left) and Juan Hernandez (below right) are renowned artists who made these trees of life.

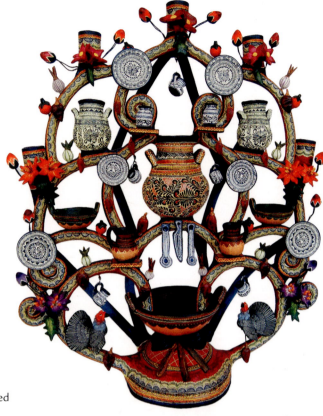

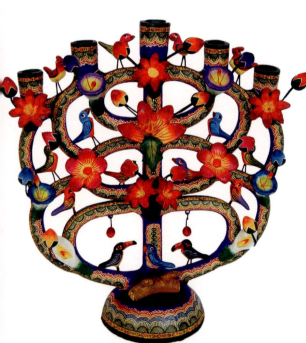

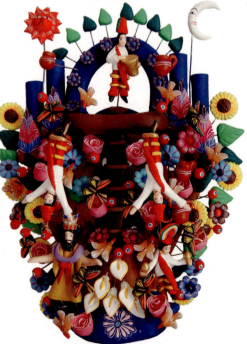

# Squash
## Calabaza
### Cucurbita moschata, Cucurbita pepo

*Cucurbita* varieties are believed to have originated in North America and belong to the same family as squash and cucumbers. They are vines with large leaves and flowers. In archeological sites in Mexico seeds have been found that date back 6000 years. Squash has been traditionally grown with corn and beans.

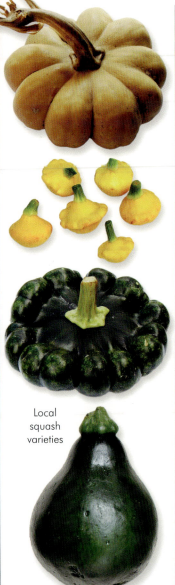

Local squash varieties

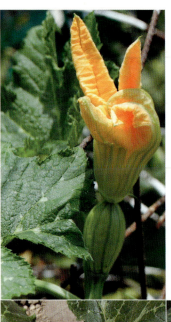

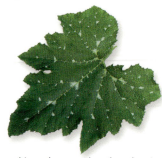

Pumpkin pulp contains vitamins A, C, potassium, and is rich in carbohydrates and proteins. Pumpkins that are yellow or orange inside are rich in beta carotene and antioxidants. Pumpkin and squash seeds have vitamin A, B, lecithin, they eliminate parasites, clean the blood vessels and stimulate kidney function. Pumpkin oil is beneficial for the heart.

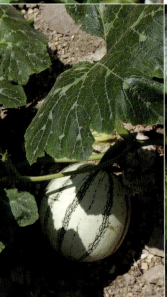

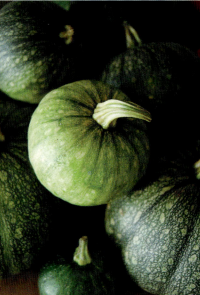

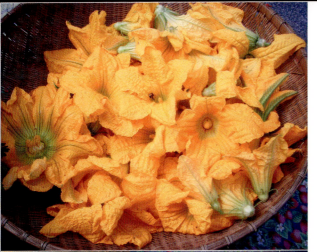
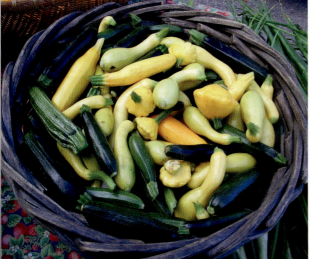
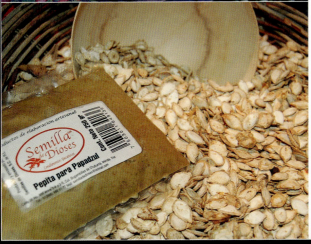

# Culinary Uses

Squash flowers are edible and are served in soups, omelets, or fried.

## Red Salsa with Chile Morita and Ground Pumpkin Seed:

Finely chopped 4 tomatos, 1 dry chile morita and a medium size onion are cooked with a little water and extra virgin olive oil until soft and mashed. Ground pumpkin seed power is mixed in until desired consistency. This salsa may be served as a dip with corn chips and vegetables or as a filling for tacos, topped with avocado and pickled red onion or any other ingredient.

## Squash with Chaya:

Cut fresh squash, onions, tomato and tender corn are fried together. When ready, finely chopped chaya leaves are added. Serve as a side dish or with rice.

## Sweet & Spiced Pumpkin:

Large wedges of pumpkin are cooked in a slow process with cane sugar and many spices during the last months of the year for seasonal festivities.

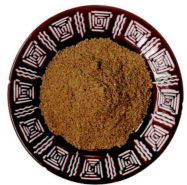

Ground pumpkin seed powder is used in many traditional dishes

Next page, left: A meal of *tortillas* with salsa and ground pumpkin seed.
Next page, right: Cream of squash soup with corn and roasted chile poblano.

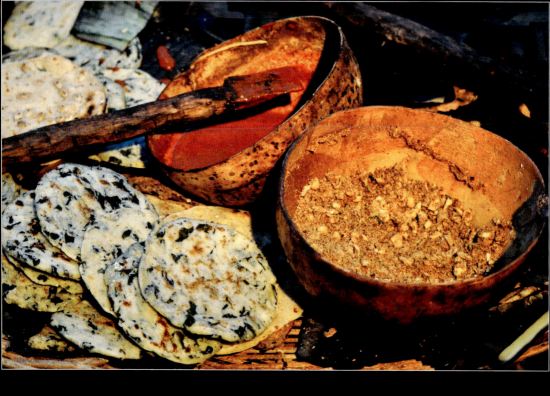

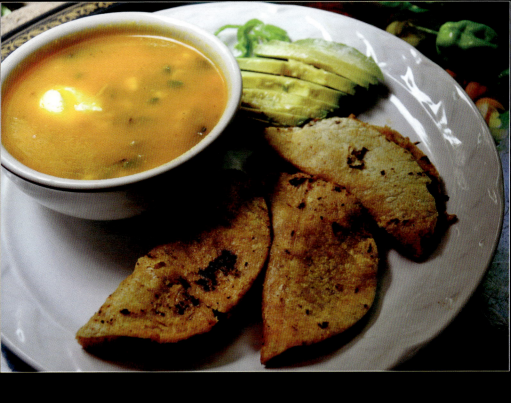

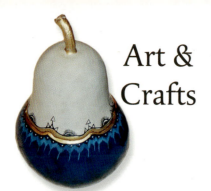

# Art & Crafts

Gourds that are common in Mexico come from a tropical tree *Crescentia Alata* or *Crescentia Cujete*. It is believed to have originated in Africa and spread to the rest of the world very early. Dried gourds are carved or painted and made into many artistic and domestic objects such as bowls, bottles, musical instruments, masks, baskets and lamps.

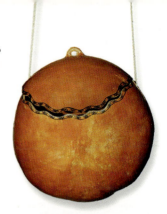

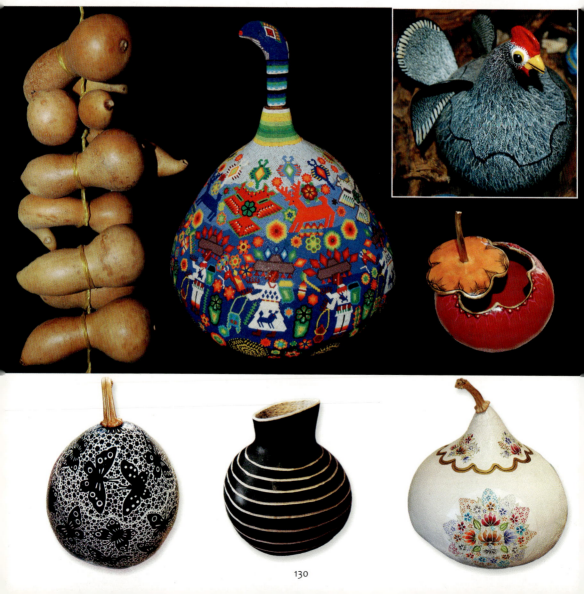

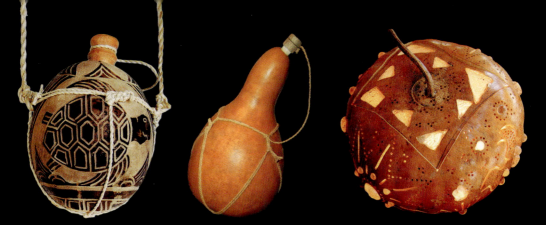

Gourds are still used as household or decorative items.

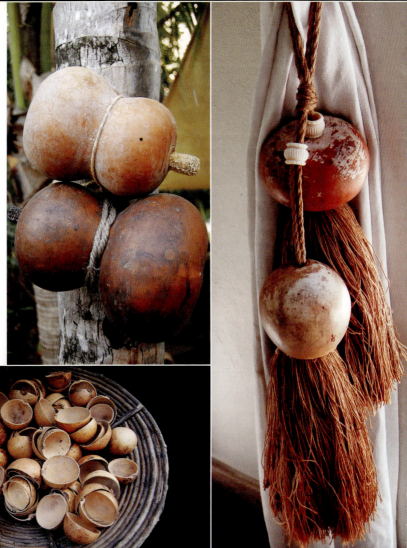

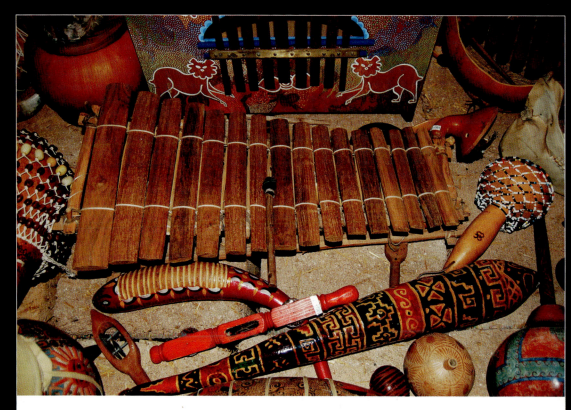

# Musical Instruments

Wind and percussion instruments were the most common in ancient Mexico. The Maya had trumpets, flutes, whistles, seashells, maracas and different types of drums. Music was an integral part of life, it was used in rituals, prayers, official festivals and family celebrations and was considered to be of divine origin. Secular music was also considered a gift from the gods, as stated in the *Popol Vuh*.

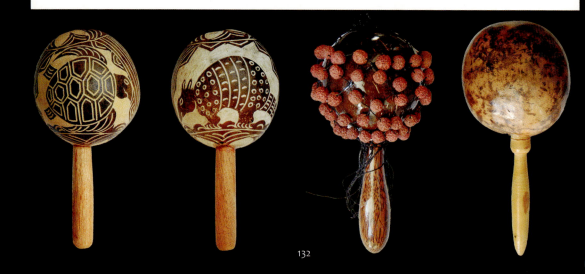

Drums were made with deerskin and played mosty with the hands or struck with a long wooden stick coated with resin on the end. Some were carved from hardwood with an H-shaped slot. Whistles were made of clay or wood and decorated with pictures of plants and animals.

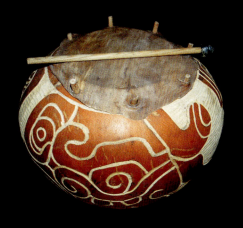
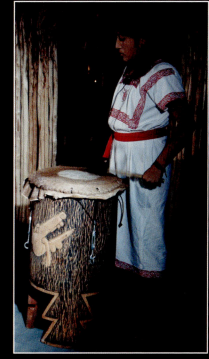
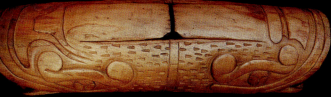
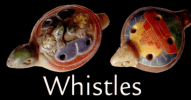

## Whistles

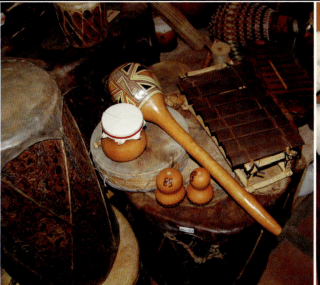
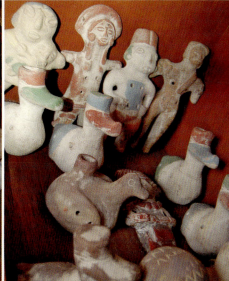

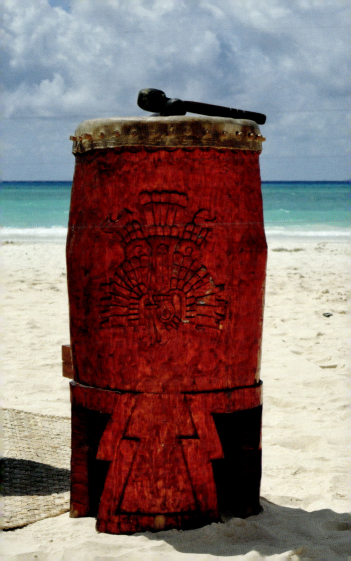

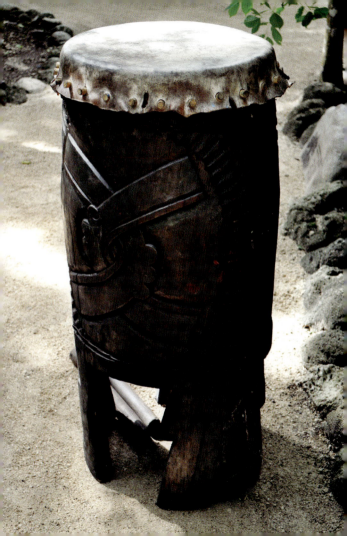

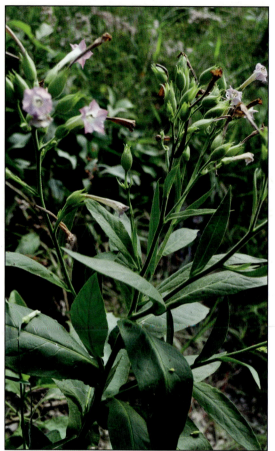

# Tobacco

## Spanish Name: Tabaco
### Scientific Name: Nicotiana tabacum
### Nicotiana rustica

For neuralgia a tincture made with 4 g of tobacco in 100 g of alcohol is strained and applied externally to the affected area.

To expel rectal parasites a rinse is prepared by boiling 1 g of leaves in 100 g of water.

As a remedy for rheumatism a tincture is prepared with 3-4 g of tobacco for 100 g of alcohol and is applied externally to the affected area.

For medicinal purposes fresh or dried tobacco leaves may be used.

The presence of a tobacco plant in a garden will keep some insects away from your crops.

Tobacco plants belong to the family of *Solanaceans* and are native to the American continents. The most common among this family and most well researched are *Nicotiana tabacum* and *Nicotiana rustica*. *Nicotiana tabacum* has relatively limited distribution because it does not adapt well in a climate other than tropical. *Nicotiana rustica* is more hardy and it has spread throughout different climate zones in many continents. For millennia tobacco was used by the Aztecs, the Incas and the Maya.

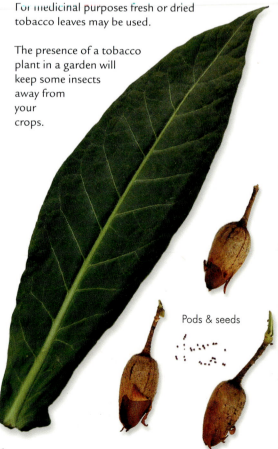

Pods & seeds

"Everything has emanations. The interactions of emanations produces new combinations. This refers to man, to the earth and the microbe."
G. I. Gurdjieff

# sacred plants

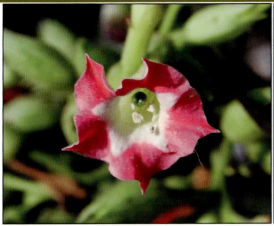
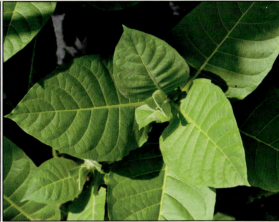

Tobacco flowers vary in color and have a pleasant smell.

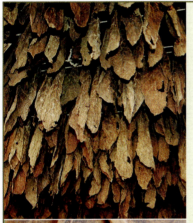

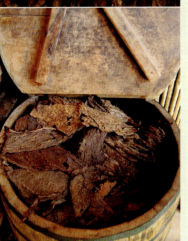

## Cigars

The traditions of tobacco use in the Americas have their roots in great antiquity. Its use was mainly confined to magic and religious purposes more than medicinal and its significance was enormous. The most common practice was to smoke the leaf, in some places to inhale it or chew, sometimes mixed with ashes or other ingredients. *Nicotina rustica* has moderately higher content of alkaloids and is a robust plant that was sold at the markets of Tenochitlan. The custom among the noble and rich Aztecs was to smoke tobacco leaves aromatized with liquid amber incense. Nicotine is the main alkaloid and toxic substance in tobacco. It is an excellent insecticide and was used as such until the introduction of organofosforados (phosphate fertilizers), which are toxic for the plants, while tobacco is not.

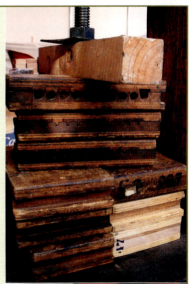

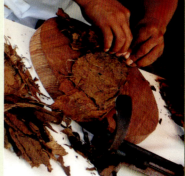

# The Sacred Calendar

Of the three Mayan codices that survived the human history the Madrid is a divination almanac, the Dresden - a compilation of astronomical and divination data and the Paris is devoted to divination in relation to certain time periods.

This evidence points to the fact that the Maya, like most other advanced civilizations of the antiquity, knew that the constellations and planets exerted their influence upon everything on earth. The knowledge of these influences was collected and developed over long periods of time and designed into a system of interlocking calendars, of which the central was *Tzolkin*, a Sacred Calendar with a 260 day cycle, consisting of time periods of 20 days. This Sacred calendar when used in combination with all the others was a basis for divination which allowed for the planning of activities on all levels of society.

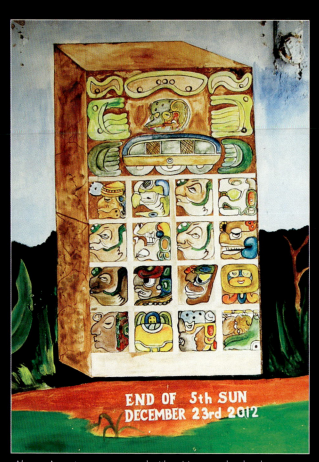

Above: A contemporary mural with a Mayan calendar theme near Valladolid, Mexico.

So precise were the calculations of the Maya, that the cycles of the three calendars, the Solar, the Sacred and the Venus – coincided every 104 years, or 2 cycles of 52 years. Chronological time keeping was done in accordance with the solar calendar of 365 years. The lunar calendar, the charts for the movements of Mars, Mercury, Jupiter and Saturn were used as part of this divination system.

It is not exactly known when, where and how the Sacred Calendar has originated, but there are theories that suggest that it may have been originally designed in Izapa, was developed to perfection by the Maya and adopted for the practical use throughout the Mesoamerica.

The relation of time and space seems to have been one of the central aspects of the Mayan science and the practical way to relate to it is depicted in the well known representation of time periods as gods bearing the burden on their backs, who, according to the carried burden, were exerting a beneficial or malevolent influence upon the earth and the people.

Consulting an astrologer-priest would determine the right time to plant the crops, or have a wedding, or give the right name to a child. To keep track of the astrological data in relation to time and space, the Maya developed a unique numbering system, which included the concept of zero.

Of all the Mesoamerican civilizations only the Maya created the science capable of projecting great lengths of time. In Palenque there is a recorded date going back 1,250,000 years. For the Maya the time was not a motion, but rather an on-going duration which assumed a constant anticipation, preparation and realization.

The ceremonies were based on the precise knowledge of the influence during a particular time period, making it favorable for the power of thought and intention to be released into space and time, followed by anticipation and work in order to turn it into a manifested realization.

The science of astrology combined with the knowledge and study of plants formed the foundation for the practice of medicine.

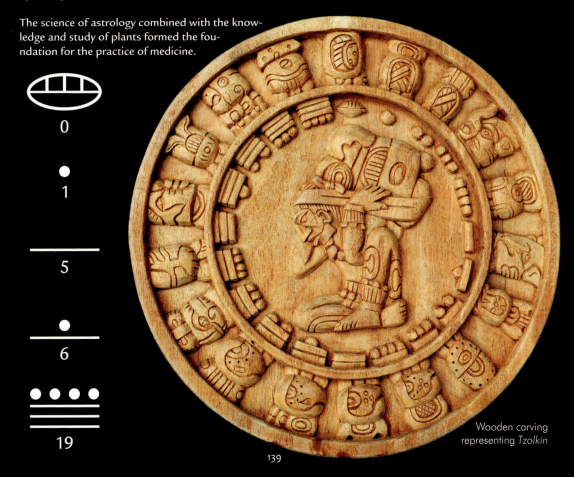

Wooden carving representing *Tzolkin*

# Verbena

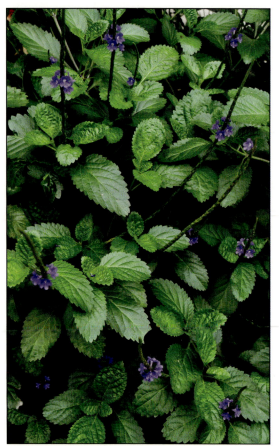

Verbena, also called vervaine, is a perennial herb about 1-2 m tall. It belongs to a genus of about 250 species of annual and perennial plants common in many continents. In the Yucatan verbena grows as a wild herb in shady areas where there is enough moisture in the soil. In traditional medicine it is regarded as a sacred plant that is used in ceremonies to clear out low-frequency energies.

"Every individual's life is intimately connected with nature. How people accommodate and adapt to the seasons and the laws of nature will determine how well they draw from the origin or spring of their lives"
Huang Di, The Yellow Emperor

## Spanish Name: Verbena
### Scientific Name: Stachytarpheta cayennensis

In case of fever 5 g of leaves are boiled in 500 ml of water until the liquid is reduced in half and then taken warm on an empty stomach for several days.

Infusion made of flowers balances, protects and detoxifies the liver, stimulates bile flow and is a good remedy for some chronic liver conditions.

A few drops of juice from fresh leaves added to a cup of hot water is taken for headaches.

Leaves in infusion taken as one cup before a meal calm the central nervous system, are beneficial for the heart, stomach pain and common colds.

To get rid of parasites 1 tsp. of juice from fresh leaves is to be taken once a day for 7 days.

Tea with fresh or dry verbena leaves, chamomile and mint is an excellent bedtime drink. Let steep for 20 minutes.

Flowers boiled in water make a nice hair rinse.

Poultice made out of boiled root may be applied directly on the affected area for ulcers, bruises and tumors.

# sacred plants

In herbal medicine verbena is regarded as a safe, natural remedy when prepared in decoctions and infusions for allergies and respiratory conditions such as the common cold or flu, asthma and bronchitis. Verbena is also very beneficial for different digestive system conditions and has anti-inflammatory properties. It is believed to be effective against intestinal and skin parasites.

In ancient Rome verbena was considered a sacred plant.

Dry verbena leaves may be sprinkled on coals as incense.

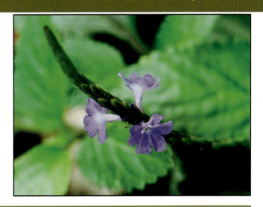

# Ixchel

*IxChel* is Goddess I of the Codices, her name means "light skinned". She is the goddess of the Moon, medicine and childbirth and the deity of everything feminine. Her energy is the force that gives fertility to the earth. She is the one who watches over the unborn children, healers and plants.

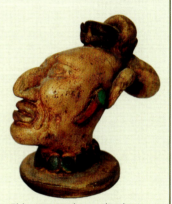

Elder *Ixchel* is depicted with a snake on her head.

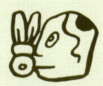

*Ix Chebel Yax*, the wife of *Itzam Na*, the lord of heavens, is the elder version of the goddess *Ixchel*. She is the one who created weaving and spinning and was the first to paint the earth red with her paint brush, so she is also the goddess of painting. Related to the Moon and medicine, she is the ruler of tides and destructive waters that become floods and tropical torments.

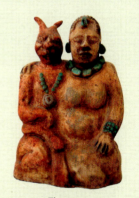

This statue represents Lunar Eclipse.

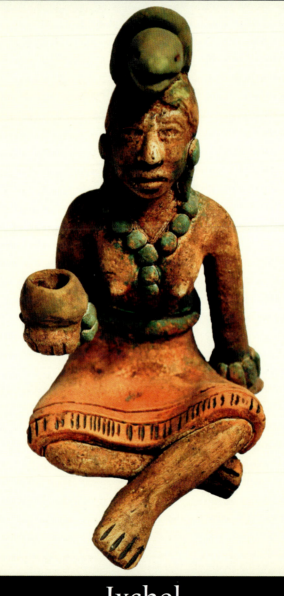

Ixchel

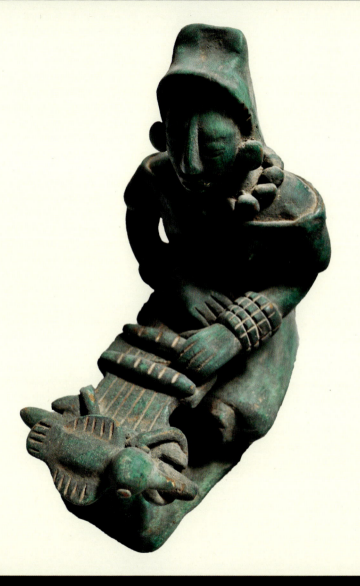

The Weaver

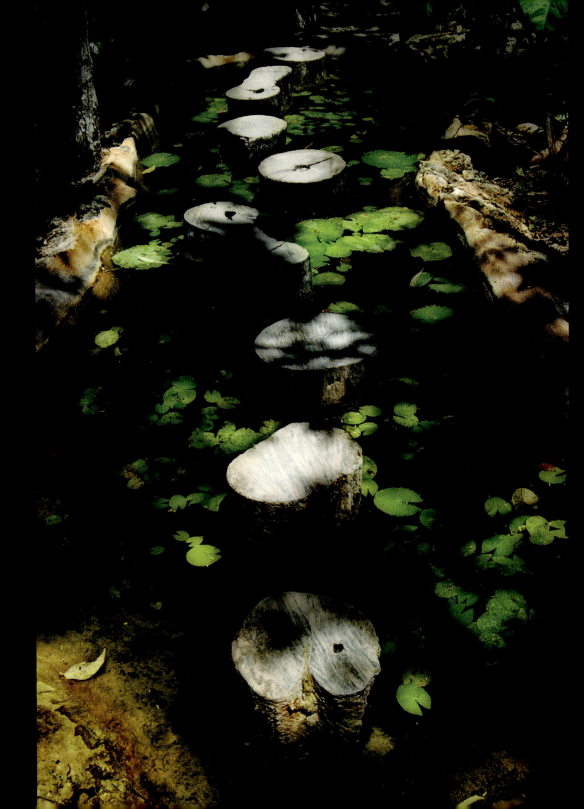

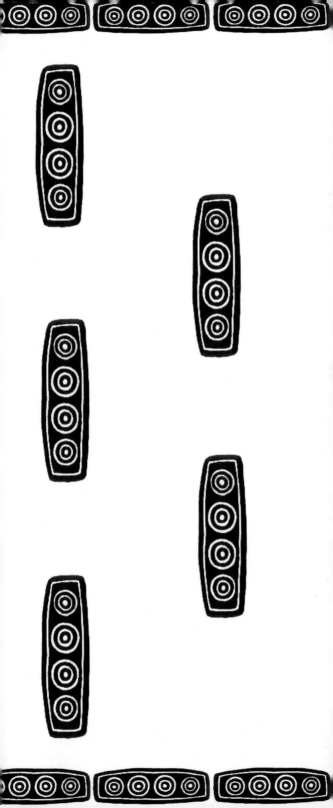

# Annato

## Spanish Name: Achiote
### Scientific Name: Bixa orellana L.

In traditional medicine annatto was used to treat some very serious conditions, including inflammation of the pleura, diabetes, tonsillitis and the oil made from the seeds was used as a remedy for leprosy.

A little annato seed powder with a few drops of vinegar in 1 glass of water helps to clear sore throat when used as a gargle after every meal.

A decoction made with seeds and a little honey is given for extreme nervous conditions and hysteria.

For diarrhea or dysentery three leaves are mashed in 1 glass of water, left to stand for a little while and then taken internally a half of a glass at a time.

For headaches leaves are applied on the temples.

For mouth sores a decoction of leaves is made and used as a rinse after every meal.

For minor burns and erysipelas an ointment is made from annato seed powder mixed with olive or grapeseed oil.

As a beauty treatment for the lips the seeds are boiled, the liquid is mixed with honey and applied for about 30 minutes, then gently washed off with water.

For infected or itching insect bites leaves are mashed in a small amount of water, left in the sun for the day and after sunset are added to the bath.

Annato is a very common tropical shrub native to American continents. It has been cultivated since ancient times for its medicinal properties and the red coloring that is extracted from its seeds. Local people used annato seeds since antiquity and now have been introduced to the rest of the world as a healthy alternative to synthetic dyes used in the cosmetic, food and textile industries.

"Intuitive logic is the highest form of both intuition and logic. It is direct knowing. This logic has one duty, and that duty is to justify intuition."
Lifting the Veil, Joseph Michael Levry

# roadside plants

Recado rojo, a paste with annato as the main ingredient, is one of the most common condiments used in Mayan cooking to season a variety of dishes. Fish marinated in annato seed and lime juice and baked with vegetables wrapped in banana leaves is a popular specialty in the Mexican Caribbean cuisine.

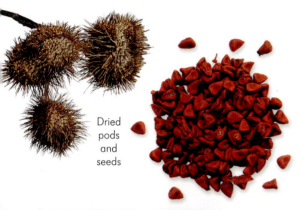

Dried pods and seeds

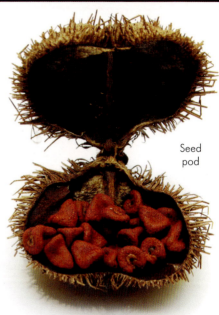

Seed pod

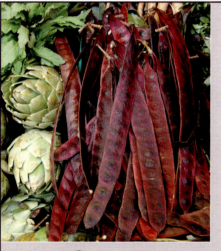

## Guaje
### Leucaena esculenta

A colorful drawing depicting the harvesting of *guaje* decorates the famous Florentine Codices of the XVI century. Its medicinal and culinary use has been well documented and it may be found in the markets throughout Mexico.

This plant is a small vine. It is used raw and cooked and may be prepared with garlic, slightly stir-fried or steamed.

The seeds, roasted tomatoes and green chiles are ground up in a *molcajete* with a little water and salt to make a delicious traditional salsa, typical for Chiapas.

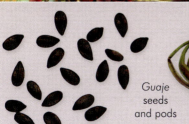

Guaje seeds and pods

# Arnica

## Spanish Name: Arníca
### Scientific Name: Arnica sp.

Arnica is widely used externally for its anti-inflammatory and pain relieving qualities. Rubbed on the skin as a cream, ointment, salve, or tincture, arnica helps to soothe muscle aches, reduce inflammation, heal wounds, acne, angina, atherosclerosis, insect bites, sprains and injuries with unbroken skin.

An infusion made of flowers and applied as a poultice is good for bruises, minor internal traumas and swellings due to sprains. Use 5 g of flowers for 1 l of water. It also serves as a muscular tonic for people active in sports; the same remedy applied on the chest area serves as a relief for bronchitis.

A decoction of 20 g of leaves boiled in 1 l of water, cooled and applied as a poultice on affected area is a good remedy for hemorrhoids.

Tincture applied on the scalp promotes hair growth.

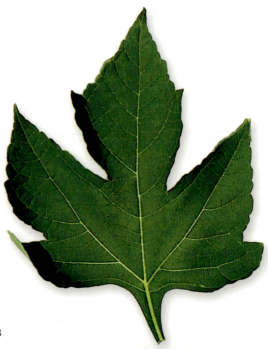

Arnica, or leopard's bane, is native to the mountains of Europe and Siberia. There are many species of this perennial plant, easily found in many parts of the world. The flowers are collected whole and dried. Preparations made from them have been used in herbal medicine for hundreds of years. The root is collected in autumn after the leaves have died down. The leaves may be used along with flowers in preparation of ointments and lotions.

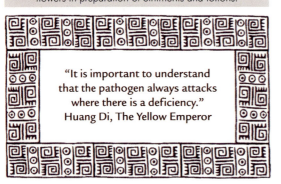

"It is important to understand that the pathogen always attacks where there is a deficiency."
Huang Di, The Yellow Emperor

# roadside plants

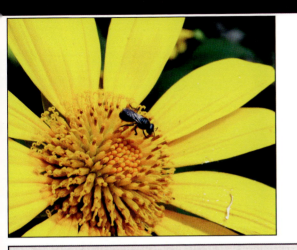

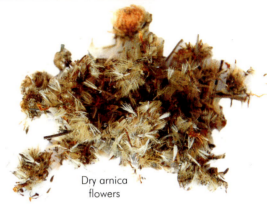

Dry arnica flowers

# Scorpion's Tail
## Cola de Alacrán
### Heliotropium indicum L.

*Cola de alacrán* is a wild growing herb common to all tropical and subtropical regions. It grows along the roads or in dry sunny spots. The small white flowers produce seeds, so there are normally a few plants growing together.

This plant has anti-septic qualities and facilitates coagulation of the blood and healing, and in case of a cut, a rinse was made with a decoction of 50 g of plant cooked in 1 l of water.

Externally this plant is a very good remedy for neuralgia, for which a paste of leaves is prepared and applied directly upon the affected area.

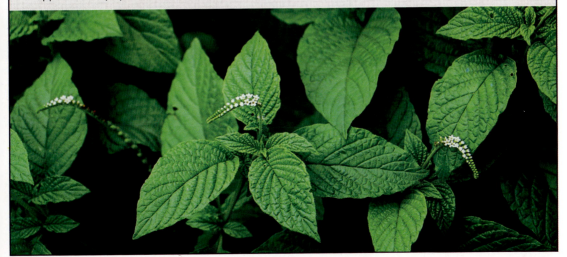

There are about half a thousand species of tropical stingless bees, of which *Melipona beeicheii* and *Melipona yucatanica* have been cultivated by the Maya for many centuries and regarded as sacred. A special ceremony was held twice a year to celebrate the harvesting of the honey. The traditional name of the Mayan stingless bee is *Xunan Kab*, which means "royal lady", and the bee god is called *Ah Muzen Cab*.

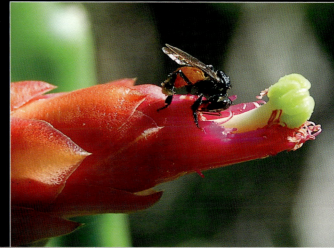

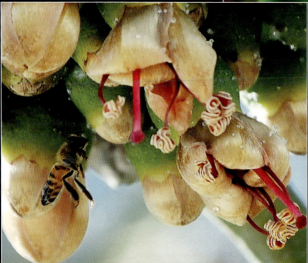

The *trigona* stingless bee (above) is twice smaller than the common African bee (left), while the *Melipona* bee is only a little smaller than the African bee. While the Mayan bees do not sting, they can bite. The *Melipona* bees have a life span of about one month, they can have up to seven queens in the same hive with virgin queens gradually leaving the beehive. *Melipona* bees work for 6 days and rest every 7th day, staying inside the beehive. *Melipona* bee hives may live up to 100 years and were passed from one generation to another.

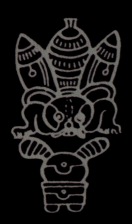

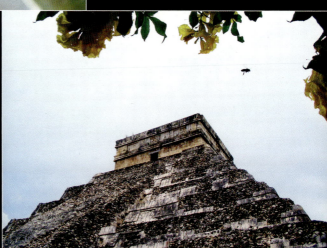

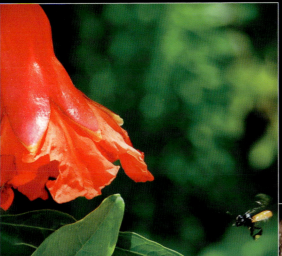

# Mayan Bee Melipona

Increasing interest in local traditions combined with an emphasis on sustainable development of the Riviera Maya, resulted in the emergence of small cooperatives that produce hilghy valued stingless bee honey. Some people pursue stingless beekeeping as a rewarding hobby. It is also fairly easy to observe the Mayan bees wherever there are flowering palm or acacia trees.

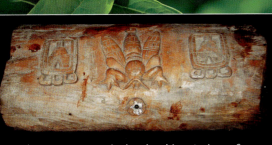

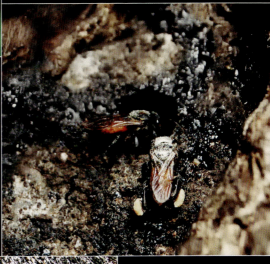

Above: A Mayan stingless bee hive. A piece of a hollow log is a good home for *Melipona* bees.
Below: Log beehives hanging on both sides of the entrance to a Mayan house.

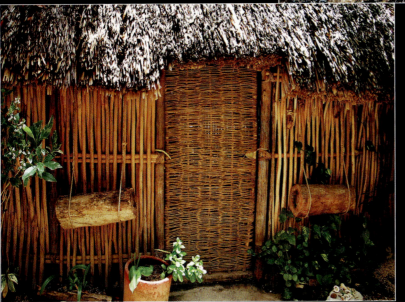

Usually a wild beehive was found in the forest in the hollow tree and a piece of the log that was holding the beehive was cut out and sealed on both ends with clay and carried to the village. There it was hung in or near the house. Honey was extracted when the seal was opened with a minimum amount of damage to the brood and pollen that are stored inside. The Mayan bee hive yields about 4-5 kg of honey per year. *Valche*, a special beverage, was prepared for this ceremony.

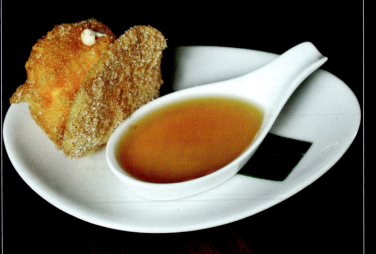

The honey from the stingless bees is also much higher in water content, which sometimes reaches up to 40%. It is almost transparent and may be a little bitter from the resin that the bees collect from the trees, to which are attributed its medicinal properties.

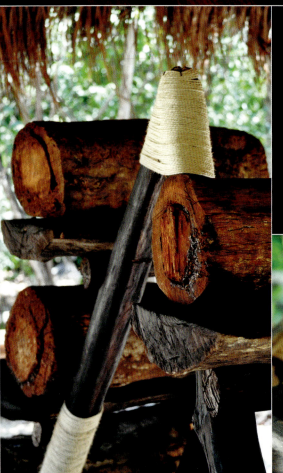

The wax made by the *Melipona* bees is soft and easy to work and was utilized in wax casting, usually popular in the bee-keeping areas. Bees were considered very special beings because upon their presence depended the harvest. In fact there are some plants that can be only pollinated by the small stingless bees and are never visited by their European or African counterparts.

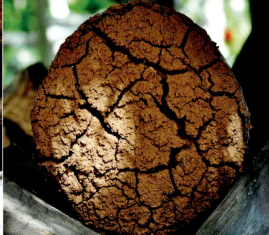

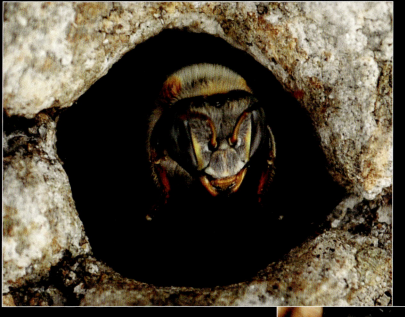

Left: Each hive has a guardian bee that oversees all incoming and outgoing traffic.

Below left: Honey is stored in balls of wax.

Below right: Honey is extracted when the balls of wax are perforated gently with a wooden stick, after which the log is tilted and the honey is poured out.

Below: The brood and the bee colony are present during the honey harvesting and remain unharmed.

Another interesting detail about these bees is that like some other animals they leave the area ahead of time if a strong natural phenomena, like a storm or hurricane, is coming. They may relocate as far as one month in advance.

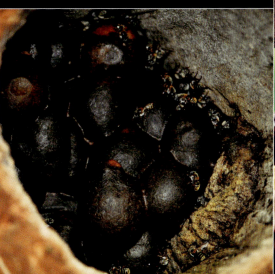

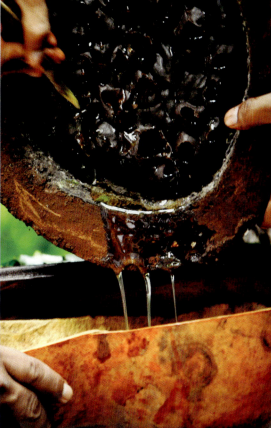

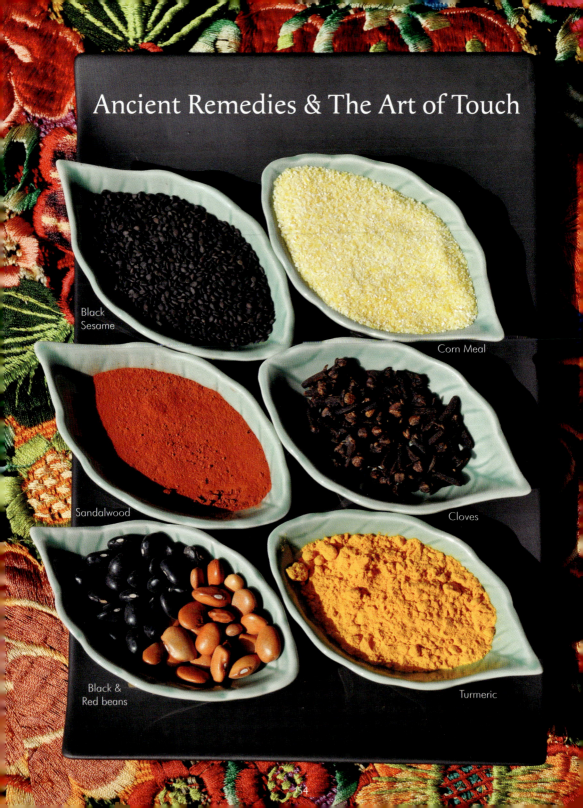

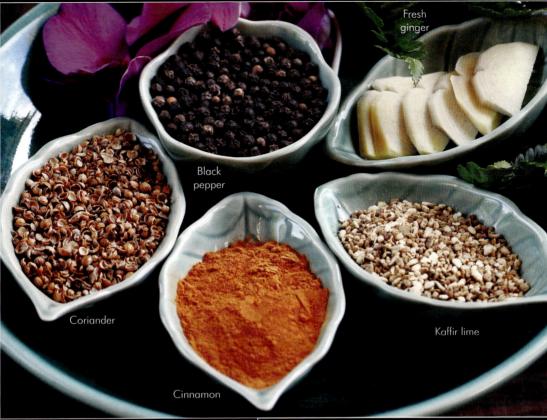

Fresh ginger
Black pepper
Coriander
Cinnamon
Kaffir lime

A holistic approach based on traditional healing therapies celebrates the human touch and the use of natural herbs and spices at the Banyan Tree Spa. Emphasis is placed on a 'high-touch, low-tech' approach and careful consideration is given to the availability and quality of all natural ingredients.

Similarities in tropical climate allow the combination of traditional Thai flavors with typical Mayan plant ingredients and create unique treatments that are available at Banyan Tree Spa Mayakoba.

Here, in support of indigenous communities and the practice of sustainable bee-keeping, the honey of the *Melipona* bee mixed with Mayan clay is used to nourish and firm the skin, leaving it soft and silky smooth after gentle application.

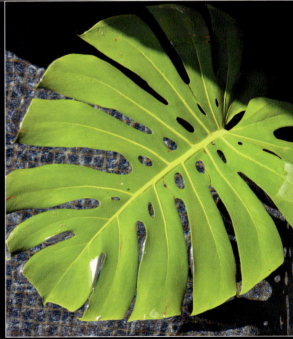

# Black Poison Wood

## Spanish Name: Chechen
## Scientific Name: Metopium brownei

*Chechen* is highly prized for its hard and tight grain wood that has very beautiful reddish-orange shades. **Sanding dust can cause dermatitis and respiratory problems, so it needs to be handled very carefully.**

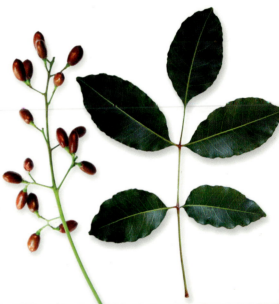

*Chechen* is a tall tree, growing up to 50 m in height. It is part of the *Anacardeiaeae* family, which also includes cashews, poison oak, poison ivy, and poison sumac. The black sap is caustic and if it comes in contact with the skin it causes a severe rash or burn and unbearable suffering, for which gumbolimbo tree bark is the best known remedy.

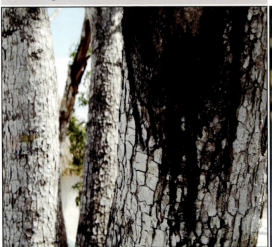

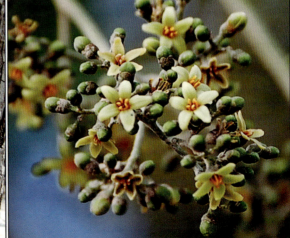

# roadside plants

# Castor Oil Plant
## Ricinus communis

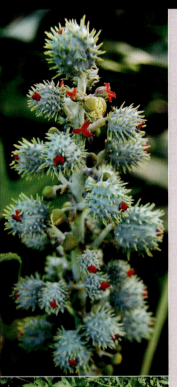

Plants are called poisonous because contact or use of them causes adverse reactions. Some plants have chemicals that we consider poisonous because they protect plants from insects. Others just accumulate substances overtime, since plants do not have excretory systems, and even though the presence of these substances is harmless for the plant itself, for animals or humans it may be harmful.

The castor oil plant is a flowering plant from the family of spurge. It has been cultivated since antiquity because the oil is slow burning and very suitable for lamps. The seeds may contain up to 60% of oil. The seed also contains a toxin, making this plant one of the most dangerous in the world. It is better to avoid handling plants that have toxicity and if it is necessary to use them medicinally, it needs to be done under the supervision of an experienced herbalist.

Castor oil has been used for body ointments, hair growth stimulating potions, as a laxative and an arthritis remedy.

There are red and white flower varieties, of which the red ones are most common in the Yucatan, growing in sunny spots and surviving with very little moisture.

Seeds and pod

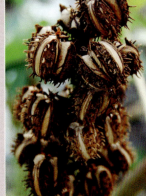

# Boat Lily

## Spanish Name: Maguey Morado
### Scientific Name: Tradescantia spathacea

Recently boat lily has been extensively studied for its medicinal properties. In traditional medicine it was used in the treatment of many skin disorders. It is believed to have decongestant, expectorant and anti-microbial properties. While the juice from the leaves is commonly applied externally, the sap from the stem is considered to be toxic.

The flower is used medicinally for the treatment of dysentery.

Extract from this plant is also used in cosmetics.

Tincture made with boat lily is being studied for its anti-tumor properties.

A beautiful perennial herb native to tropical Americas, very widely spread in forests and urban areas. In the Yucatan there are two varieties, one taller than the other. Both have similar leaves and small white flowers. Boat lily has diverse reproductive functions and grows where soil is poor and dry or on rocks. It spreads very quickly and if not controlled it may prevent other plants from growing.

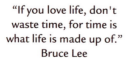

"If you love life, don't waste time, for time is what life is made up of."
Bruce Lee

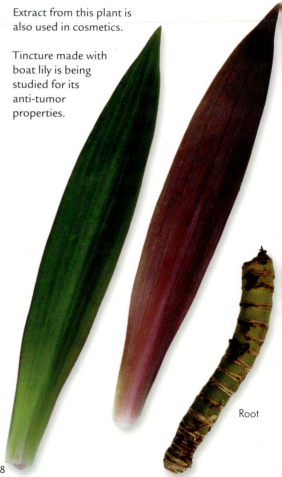

Root

# roadside plants

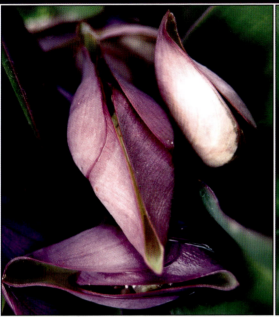
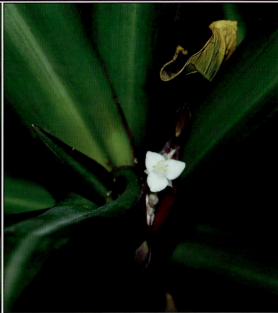

## Miracle Leaf
### Siempre Viva
#### Kalanchoe gastonis bonnieri

Miracle leaf is a small plant usually about 50-80 cm tall with thick and juicy leaves. It originated in Madagascar and is easily recognized because it forms new plants on the edges of the leaves. Goethe was passionately fond of this plant and liked to give its babies as gifts. He discussed its properties in the essay "History of My Botanical Studies". It is sometimes called Goethe's Plant.

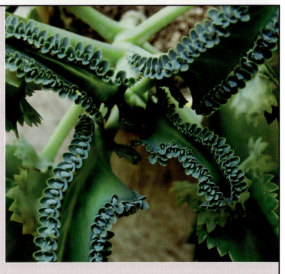

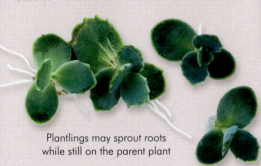

Plantlings may sprout roots while still on the parent plant

Mashed leaves applied externally are a remedy for minor headaches, contusions, swellings and bruises. When mashed with castor oil the leaves are a good remedy for mastitis when applied externally as a poultice.

*The flowers of some species are poisonous.*

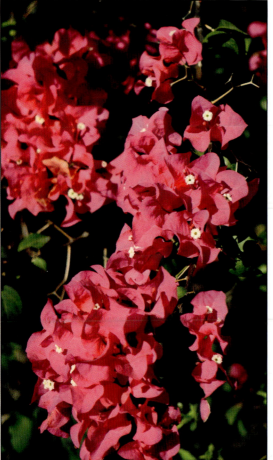

# Bougainvillea

## SPANISH NAME: BUGANVILIA
### SCIENTIFIC NAME: BOUGAINVILLEA GLABRA

Only the pink flowers are used for respiratory conditions, usually in combination with other herbs.

A tincture of the pink flowers in combination with mango buds, sauco, eucalyptus and gordo lobo can be beneficial for asthma.

An infusion of 2 g of young leaves in 100 ml of water, sweetened with honey and taken 3 times a day is a good remedy for cough.

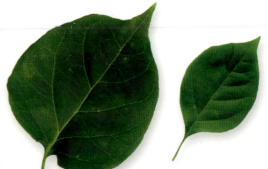

Bougainvillea grows in subtropical and tropical climates. It is common in forests where it can attach itself to other plants in order to reach sunlight. It can spread very quickly, and can be grown from clippings. It is almost insect-free because its thorns protect it. This plant can reach over 10 m in height and may grow as a vine, tree, or shrub. Bougainvillea varies in color and is frequently used as an ornamental plant that bears flowers all year.

 "Extreme grief can damage the lungs, but may be counteracted by the emotion of happiness." Huang Di, The Yellow Emperor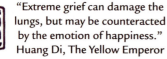

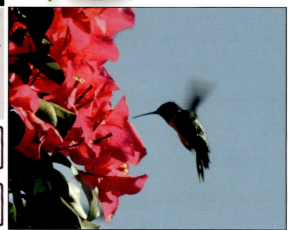

The Bougainvillea was discovered by a French botanist named Philibert Comerson in the late 1760's in Rio de Janiero and named after the captain of their ship, Louis Antoine de Bougainville.

# roadside plants

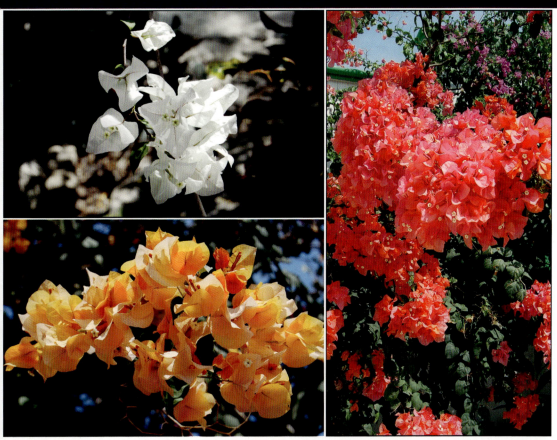

Above: Decorative bougainvilleas are not used medicinally.

# Golondrina
## Euphorbia

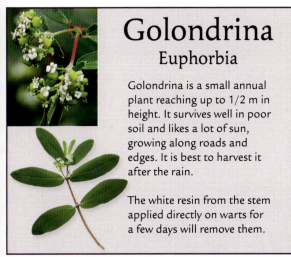

Golondrina is a small annual plant reaching up to 1/2 m in height. It survives well in poor soil and likes a lot of sun, growing along roads and edges. It is best to harvest it after the rain.

The white resin from the stem applied directly on warts for a few days will remove them.

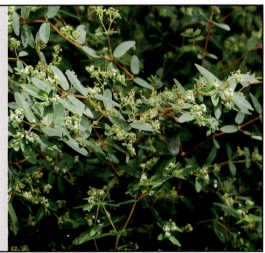

# Bromeliads

Bromeliads constitute a very large family of plants with over 3000 varieties. Many species are native to Central and South America. Bromeliads are epiphytes; they attach themselves to another living plant without taking any of the host plant's resources or affecting it in any adverse way. Some bromeliads absorb moisture from the air, while others preserve dew and rain water in the rosette formed by their leaves.

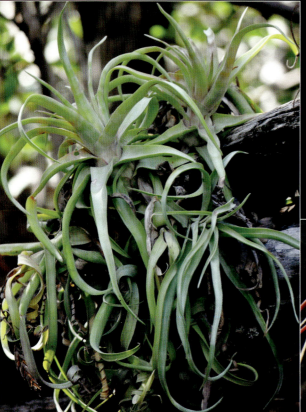

Insects, birds and small mammals often come to drink from the bromeliad leaves. Some species develop root systems, while others rely entirely upon the aerial parts for their nourishment.

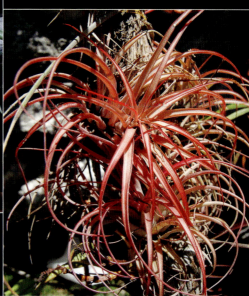

Wild growing bromeliads in the selva of the Caribbean coast.

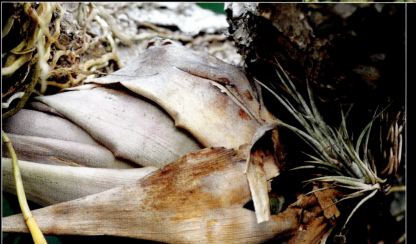

Bromeliads are very adaptable and grow well in the tropical forests of the Yucatan Peninsula and at the elevation of 4000 m above sea level in Peru.

# Decorative varieties

Bromeliads have been the favorites of tropical gardeners for a long time. Some decorative varieties adapt well to the indoor climate of the more temperate climate regions. The stalk and flowers are usually very bright and exotic looking, which makes the bromeliad a popular decorative plant. Some flowers last for a very long time, changing their color during the blooming period.
The bromeliads of Xcaret are shown here and on the following two pages.

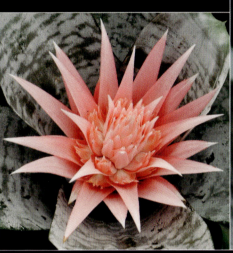
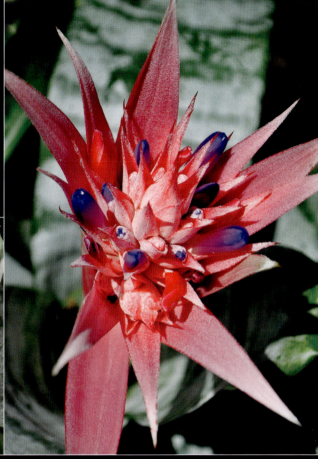

# Pineapple
## Piña
### Ananas comosus

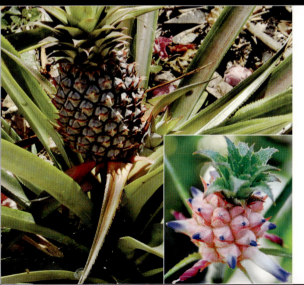

When the pineapple ripens on the plant the amount of sugar doubles in the last stage. If harvested when green they never reach this peak. Pineapples improve digestion, and fresh juice is excellent to take before meals; pineapple juice with black pepper helps to restore the electromagnetic field after using computer. Pineapple is high in vitamin C, A and B, papain enzyme, and is beneficial for anemia and rheumatism. The pineapple is one of the most known members of the bromeliad family.

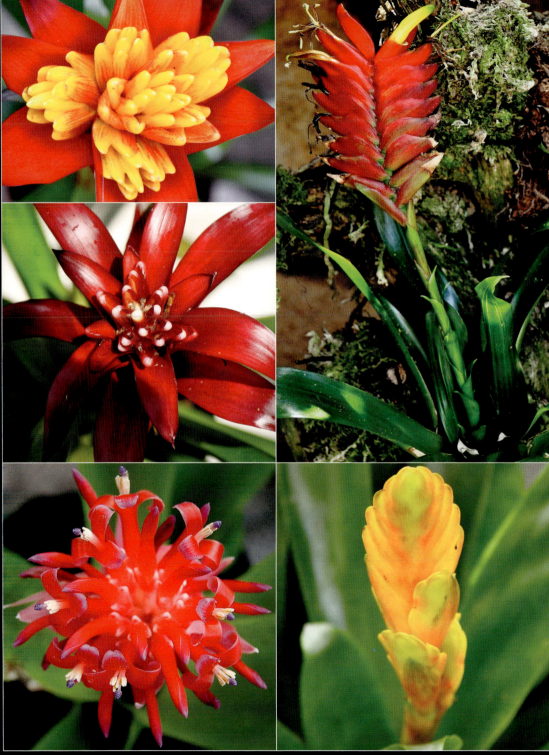

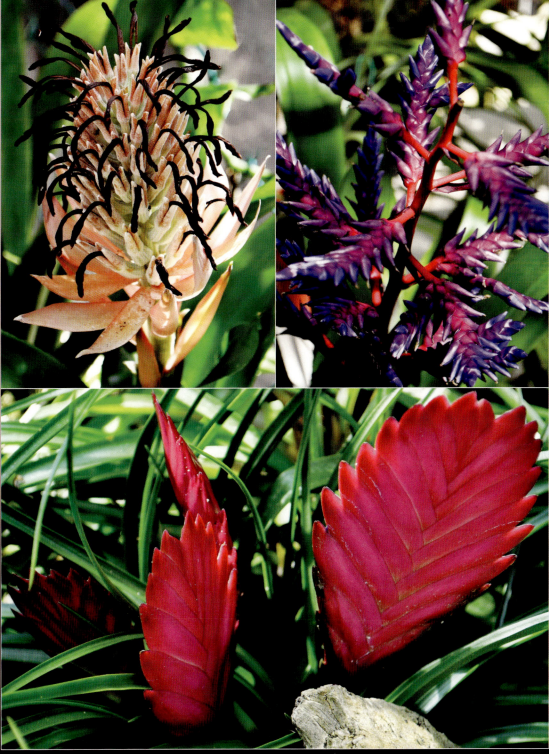

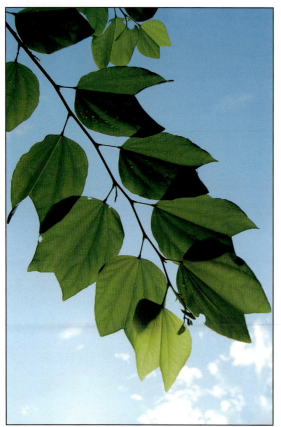

# Bull Hoof

## Spanish Name: Pata de Vaca
### Scientific Name: Bauhinia divaricata L.

Bull hoof was used traditionally as a tonic that balances and strengthens overall body function and has diuretic and expectorant properties.

Usually the leaves are harvested and used fresh or are dried to be used in infusions.

The bull hoof flowers are very beneficial in infusions for the respiratory system. They can be combined with hibiscus and bougainvillea flowers to make herbal tea to take for colds and chest congestion. Warming spices such as ginger or cinnamon may be added to the above recipe. It is always better to use honey or other natural sweetners, such as agave or maple syrup with herbal teas and infusions.

Bull hoof leaves and tea bags are common items on pharmacy shelves in South America; traditionally a dry leaf tea or infusion is enjoyed after every meal to help the body balance sugar levels.

Bull hoof grows as a small tree or vine usually not taller than 5-9 m. Its leaves are 7-10 cm long and shaped like a bull hoof, which is distinctive to the *Bauhinia* genus. It is common in Mexico and can be found in the rainforests and tropical parts of Central and South America as well as in tropical zones of Asia.

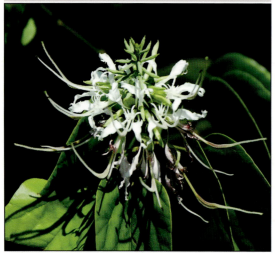

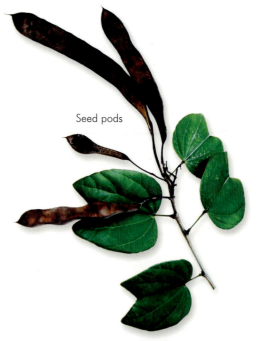

Seed pods

# roadside plants

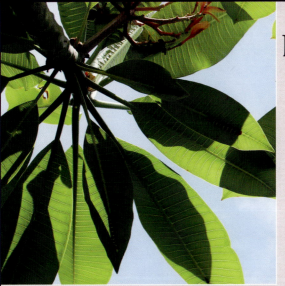
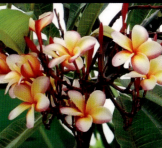
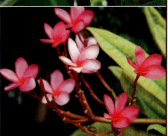

## Pogodo Tree

### Flor de Cuervo

*Plumeria rubra* L.

The pogodo tree, usually not more than 10-12 m tall, is believed to have originated in India where it is commonly planted in temple gardens for the beauty of its foliage and flowers. In Mexico it grows as a smaller tree out in dry and sunny spots. The flowers are very fragrant and colors vary from white to deep pink. The leaves grow at the end of the branches. The branches break off very easily and may be planted immediately. Broken branches give white latex, which mixed with coconut oil is a local topical remedy for itching. In traditional medicine flowers, root, leaves, bark and latex are used for a wide variety of conditions. It is best to collect it during the rainy season which lasts from May to November. A poultice of steamed leaves is used as a remedy for minor swellings. A decoction of leaves added to a foot bath helps to soothe cracks and eruptions on the soles of the feet.

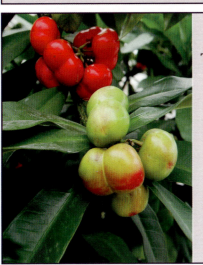

## Sanango
### *Tabernaemontana* spp.

Most species of this family are shrubs that grow up to 5-7 m in height and are used as ornamental plants throughout the Yucatan. In South America many species are used medicinally and some in combination with *ayahuasca* so that the visions can be retained and not forgotten.

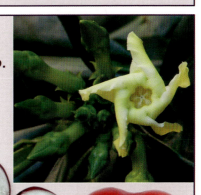

# Century Plant

## Spanish Name: Henequen
### Scientific Name: Agave fourcroydes

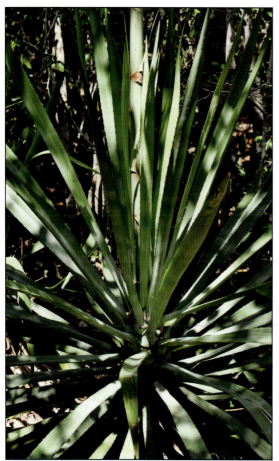

Usually it takes about 4 years for the plant to grow and mature and that is when the harvesting of the lower leaves begins. About 200 leaves can be collected off the plant before it flowers. A flower stalk can be 8 to 10 m tall with a cluster of small yellow flowers. They produce large quantities of nectar and attract a lot of bees. Agave plants can reproduce from the seeds or sprout new baby plants at the base of the parent plant.

Juice from one roasted blade of *Agave chelem* was traditionally used for asthma and other minor respiratory conditions.

Resin from the lower parts of the leaves has been used in native dentistry for tooth ache: a small piece was inserted to cover the cavity.

**This plant can be irritating and poisonous due to a high content of saponin.**

Below and opposite page: Flowers of the *Agave fourcroydes*

The agave plant has been used by the people of Central America for many thousands of years. There are many varieties of agave of which some are used only as decorative plants, while others are an important part of the economy of several states. In Mexico many types of agave are called maguey. In the Yucatan Peninsula one can still find *Agave augustifolia*, which is considered to be a wild ancestor of *Agave fourcroydes* and *Agave sisalana*. Sisal fibers are extracted from *Agave sisalana*, while henequen fibers from *Agave fourcroydes*, a plant native to Yucatan and grown commercially mainly in Mexico. *Sisal* is stronger, while *henequen* is very tough and resilient. Both were used by the Maya. Fishing nets, baskets, bags, hammocks, crude cloth and alfombras, rough rugs, are still made in small workshops around Merida.

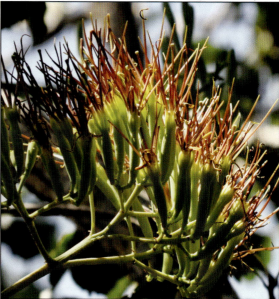

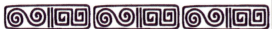

"Above all things, reverence yourself."
Pythagoras

# roadside plants

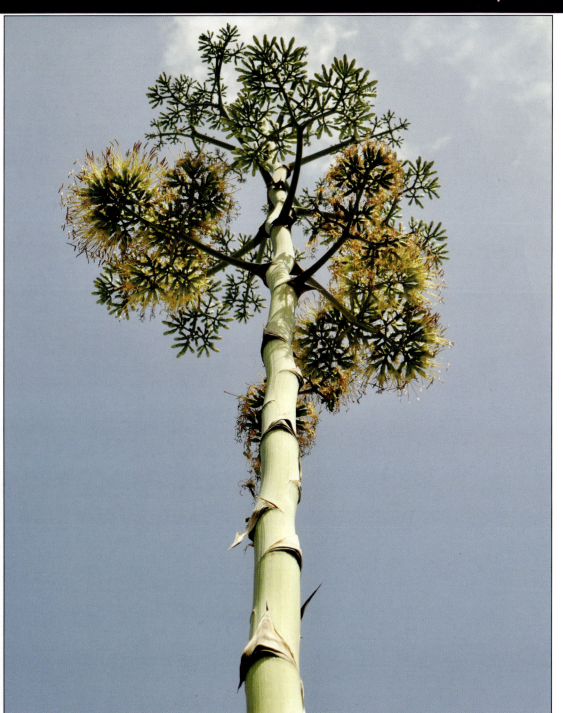

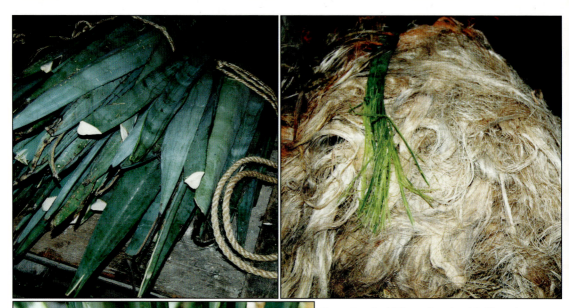

Extracting the high quality, durable fibers is an extremely labor-intensive process. *Henequen* was called the green gold of Yucatan. It is still produced commercially throughout the Yucatan Peninsula.

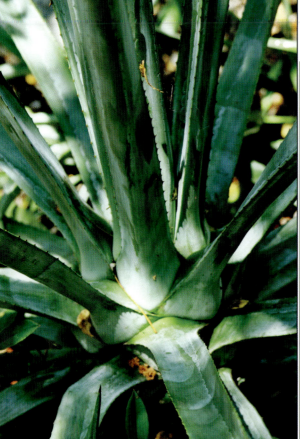

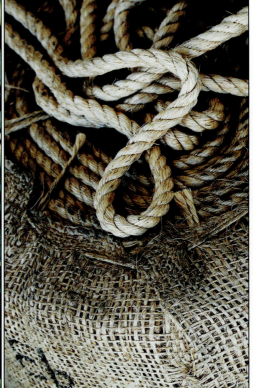

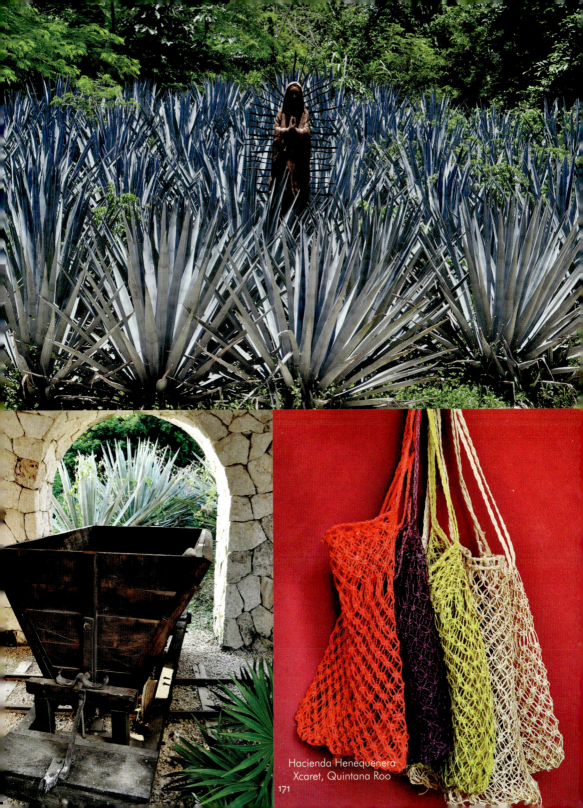

Hacienda Henequenera
Xcaret, Quintana Roo

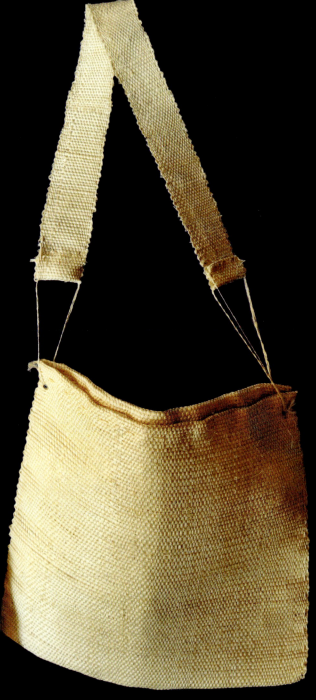

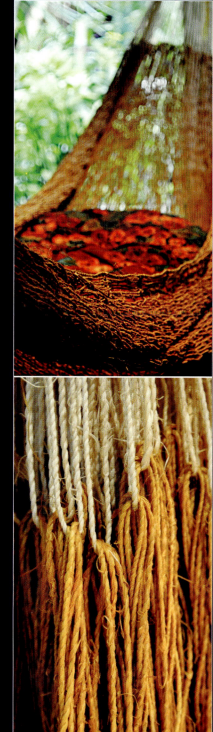

Above: Traditional Yucatecan head-bag made of *henequen* fibers.

Right: *Henequen* hammocks, a long time Yucatan specialty, may last for many years. The fibers soften with every wash.

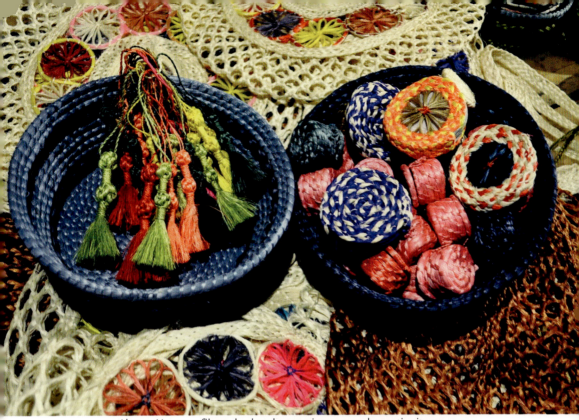

Above: *Henequen* fibers dyed and woven into many decorative items.

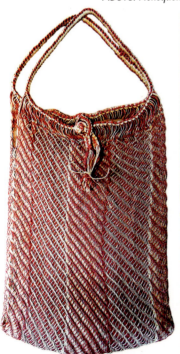

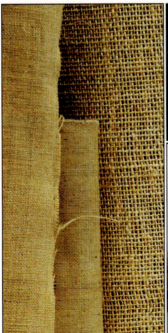

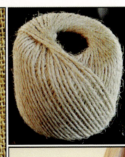

The durability and natural look of sisal makes it a popular material in arts, crafts and construction.

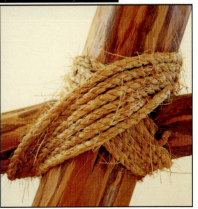

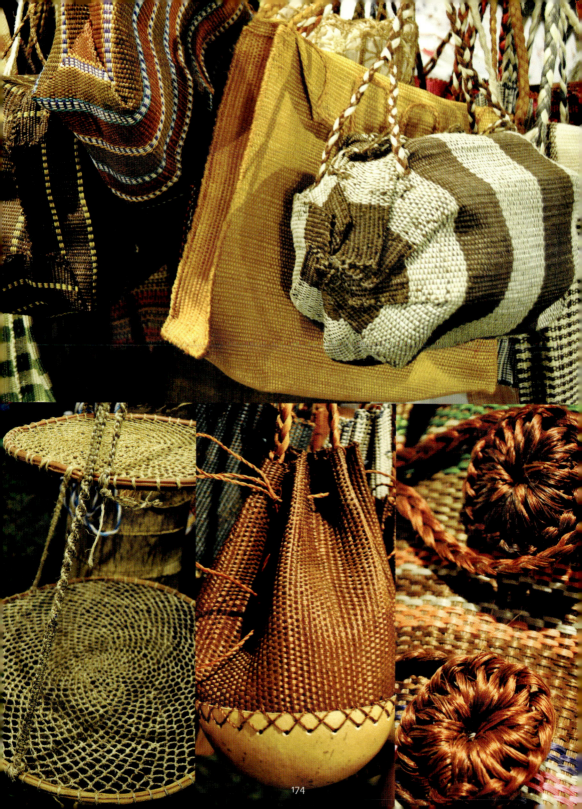

# Henequen Bags

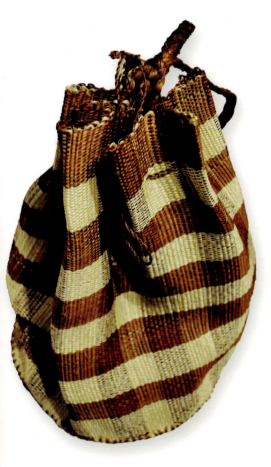
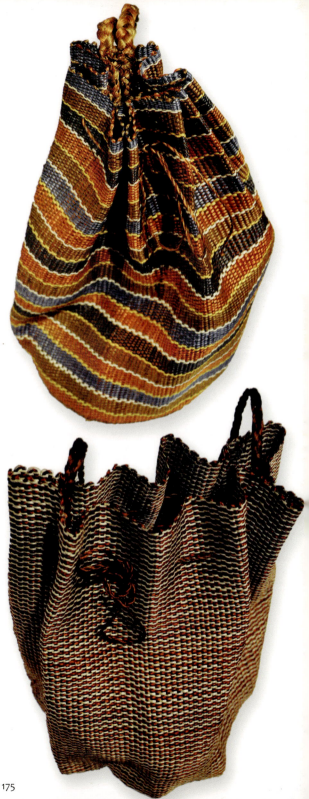

Beautiful *henequen* bags are sold at the Sunday market in the ancient town of Zaci, now knwn as Valladolid. Fiber strands, dyed with natural pigments, are woven on the shoulder strap loom, mostly by women.

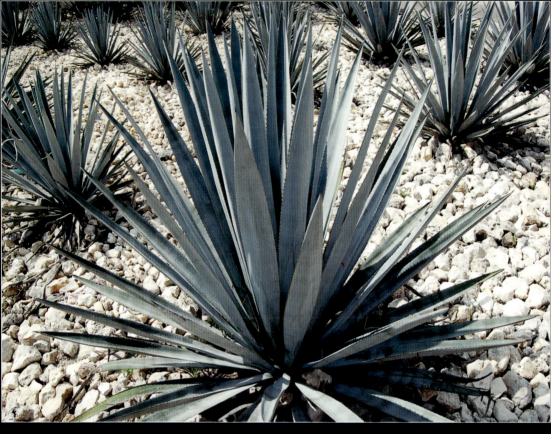

The blue agave, *Agave Tequilana* (above), is famous because it is the plant from which tequila is made. *Agave Tequilana* and related species were cultivated due to their high concentration of polysacharides. Tequila was produced by fermenting and distilling the juice from the heart of the plant. It takes about 10-12 years for the plant to mature before it can be used and by then the heart of the plant can weigh from 40 to 100 kg. The heart of the plant is heated to allow for the better extraction of the sap.
If the flower stem, or *quiote,* is cut before flowering, a sweet liquid called *agua miel* or "honey water" is collected in the heart of the plant for 6-8 months. After that the plant dies and all the remaining parts of it are used. When *agua miel* is fermented a drink called *pulque* is made, and when distilled, mezcal is produced. Mezcal is the final result of distilling the trunk, or pineapple, of the *Agave Mezcalero,* which was first cooked in an earthen oven lined with stone. This is why mescal has a smoky earthy flavor, with its strong aroma and 40% alcohol content.

There is a mescal into which the red maguey worm *(Hypopta Agavis)* is added during the bottling process to alter its flavor and color. Called *chilocuiles,* these catepillars are considered a nutricious regional delicacy when braised or deep fried and served with *tortillas* complimented by a spicy sauce.
Both mescal and tequila can be used for making herbal tinctures.

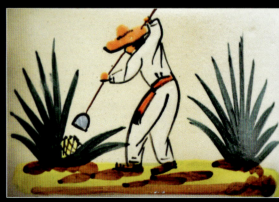

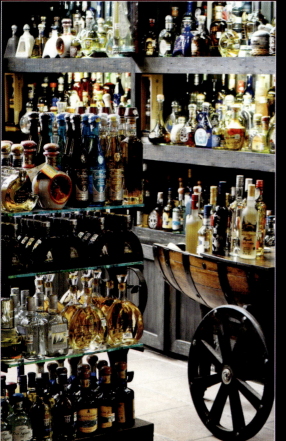

Right: Two varieties of agave syrup: dark- *miel de maguey* with strong flavor, and light- *miel de agave azul* with very pleasant and delicate flavor. Both are excellent natural sweeteners.

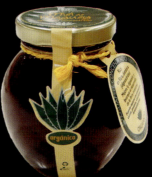
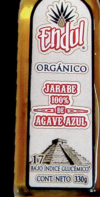

Left: *Agave azul* is very common in Jalisco and Guanajuato, where most of the tequila is produced. There are three types of tequila: *blanco*, or white, bottled inmediately after distillation, and the aged types, *reposado* and *añejo*, kept in wooden barrels for different periods of time.
Below: *Agave americana* is widely used as a decorative plant throughout the Yucatan Peninsula.

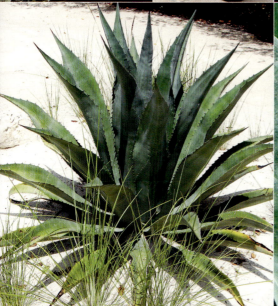
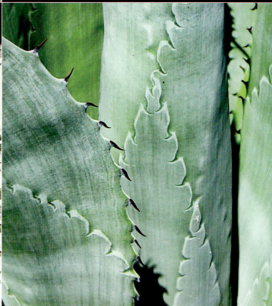

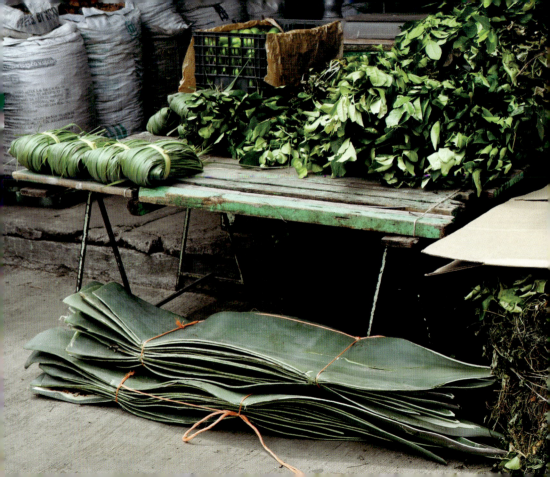

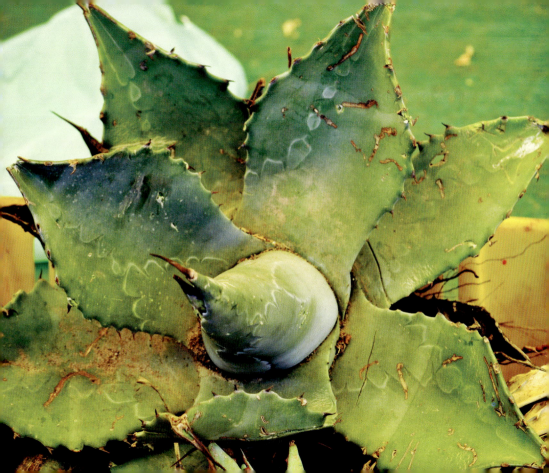

# Cotton
## Algodón
### Gossypium herbaceum

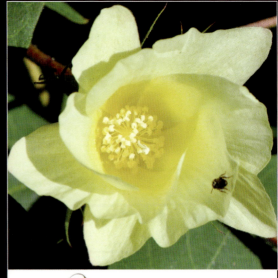

Cotton is a shrub that has been cultivated in India for 5000 years and is believed to have been brought to the New World by Europeans relatively late. Now different varieties of cotton grow in the Yucatan Peninsula, some with very rough and others with very fine fibers. Cotton also has ornamental and medicinal uses. The flowers are yellow when they first open and turn pink the following day. Cotton root and bark were known as female medicine since antiquity, while the seeds were used as a source of oil.

Cotton plants thrive in well irrigated and sunny spots.

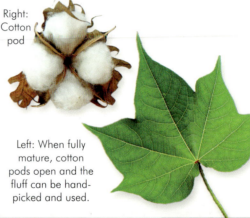

Right: Cotton pod

Left: When fully mature, cotton pods open and the fluff can be hand-picked and used.

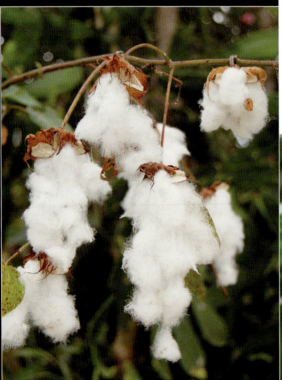

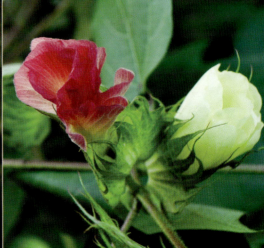

# Textiles

Since ancient times native Mexican civilizations produced a wealth of textile art. Fabrics were woven mainly from cotton and *henequen* or agave fibers. Textiles were woven on a waist loom, still seen today in the central and southern states known for their rich handicraft traditions, such as Michoacan, Hidalgo, Oaxaca, and Chiapas. People were also experts in dying cloth using many natrural ingredients of mineral, animal and plant origin. Plant based dyes were extracted from flowers, fruit, seeds, moss, bark, and wood.

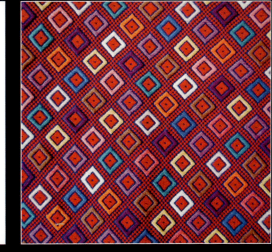
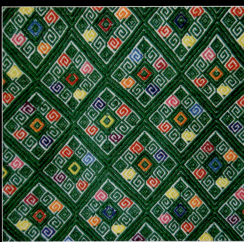
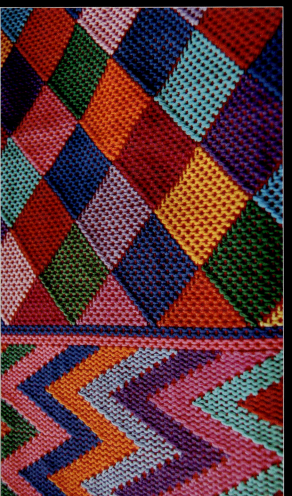
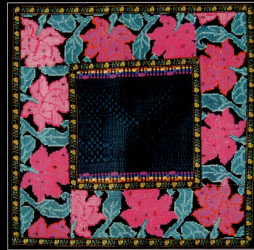

# Weaving & Embroidery

The climate conditions of Central America did not allow for the preservation of ancient fabrics, but the beauty and finesse of indigenous textiles was recorded in many chronicles. Sewing and weaving were the activities done by women. *Ixchel,* the goddess of new moon and fertility, was also considered to be a patron of *tejedoras,* or weavers.

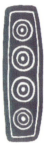 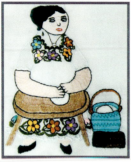 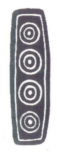

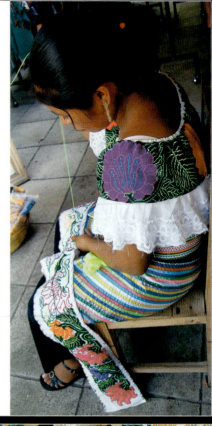

The most common Mayan women's garment is the *huipil,* worn with a fustan and *jubon.* The *huipil,* a dress of white *manta,* or cotton cloth, decorated with a bright embroidery of flowers around the neck and hem, is still worn throughout the Yucatan Peninsula. Traditionally they are washed with a bit of ash to keep them immaculately white.

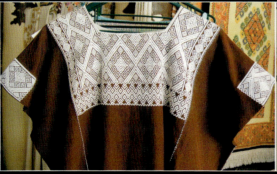 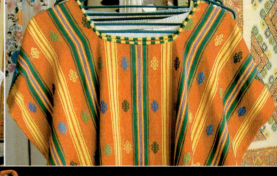

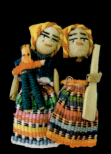 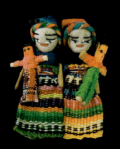 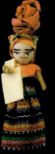 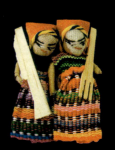 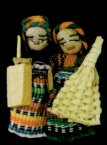

# Hammock
## Hamaca

The Yucatan Peninsula is famous for its hammocks. Originally they were made from *sisal,* bark, and palm leaves. Now hammocks are hand woven by men or women on a loom. They are still in wide use for relaxation or sleep and a family home will usually have several hammocks hung across the common room. Recent variations such as chair hammocks may be used in any modern interior.

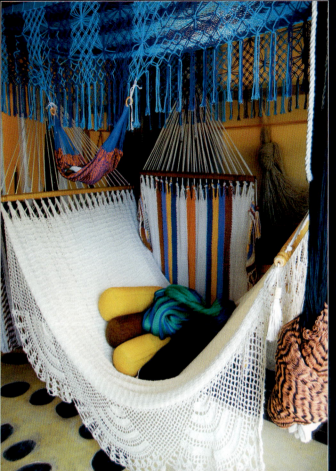

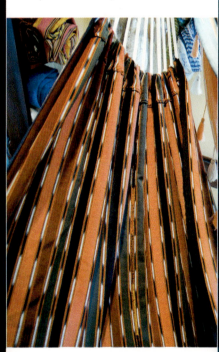

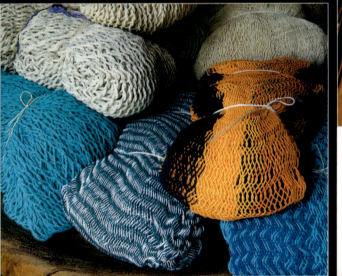

Above left: Crocheted hammocks. Hammocks are believed to have been introduced to Europe from the American continent.

Left: Most modern hammocks are made from cotton or nylon.

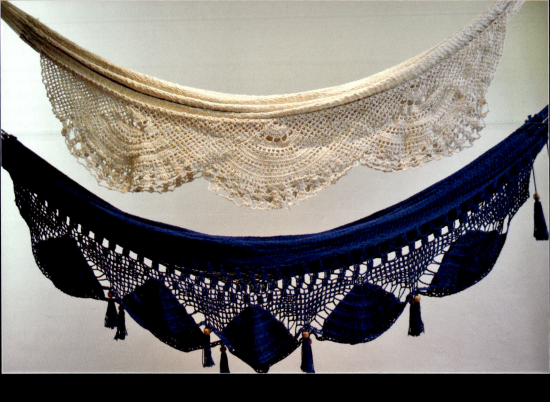

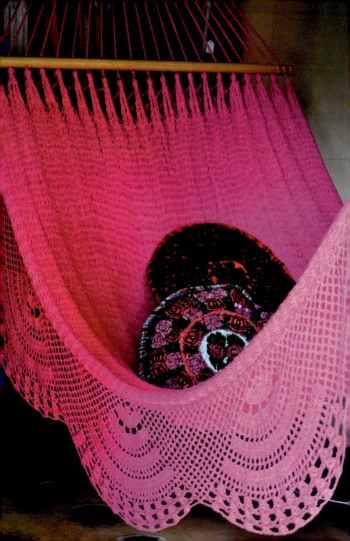

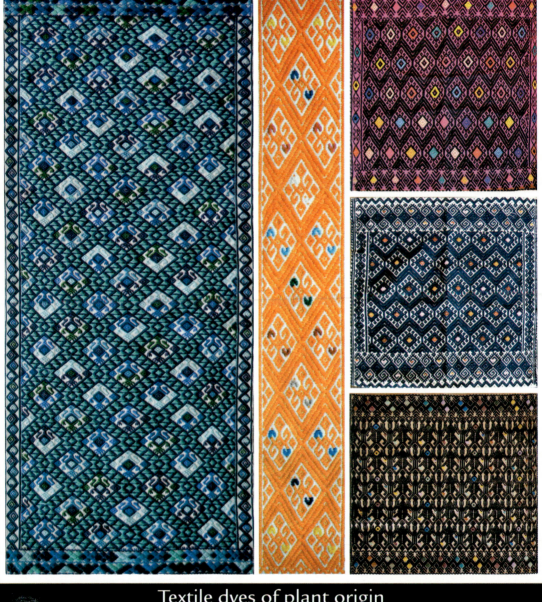

## Textile dyes of plant origin

| Orange | Blue | Brown | Gray | Yellow | Bright Red | Pink |

Orange: Annato - *Achiote* - *Bixa orellana bixácea*
Blue: Indigo - *Añil* - *Indigófera tinctoria Leguminosa*
Brown: Encino colorado - *Quercus crassifolia*
Grey: *Sacatina* - *Acantácea tinctoria*
Yellow: *Zacatlaxcalli* - *Cuscuta tinctoria Convulvulácea*
Bright red: *Palo de Brasil* - *Haematoxylon brasiletto*
Pink: *Palo de Campeche* - *Haematoxylon Campechianum*

# Huipil

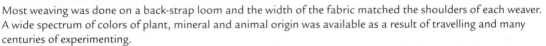

Most weaving was done on a back-strap loom and the width of the fabric matched the shoulders of each weaver. A wide spectrum of colors of plant, mineral and animal origin was available as a result of travelling and many centuries of experimenting.

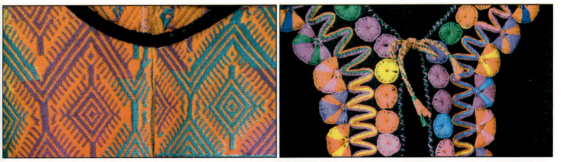

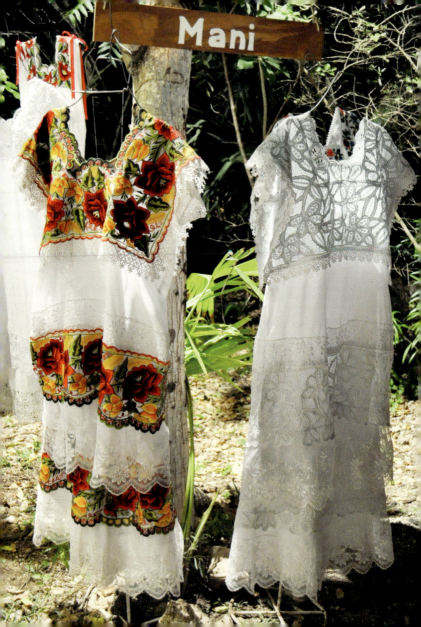

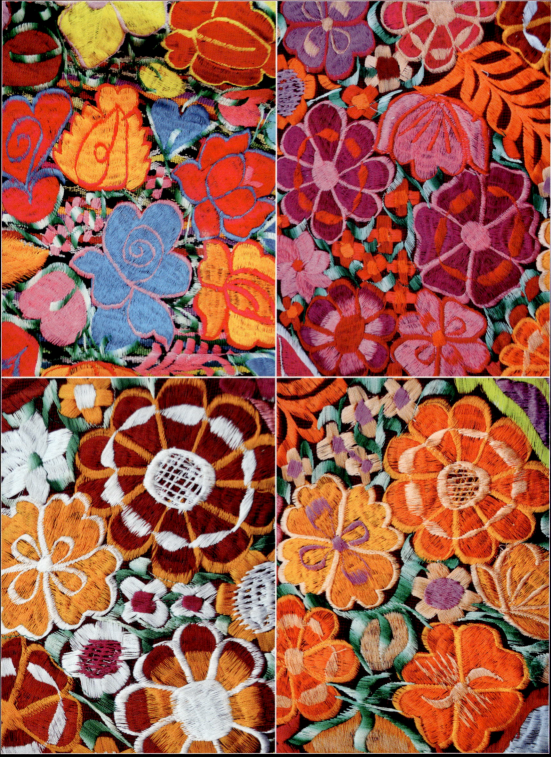

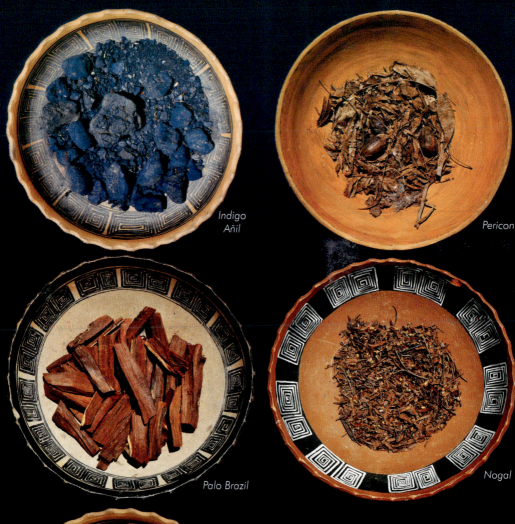

Indigo Añil

Pericon

Palo Brazil

Nogal

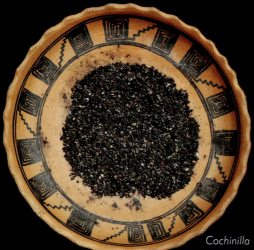

Cochinilla

# Textile dye origins

As a result of trade, traveling and many years of experimentation, a wide spectrum of colors was available for dying and each had its religious and ceremonial meaning.
 A dozen of different shades of carmine were created from *cochinilla (Dactylopius coccus)*, a small insect parasite that lives on the leaves of the nopal cactus. Brushed off and turned into powder, they were mixed with different agents to result in most amazing shades from soft pink to lemon vanilla. Orange came from the seeds of *achiote*, also used as a food seasoning. Fermented and specially prepared leaves of anil gave a deep indigo blue color.

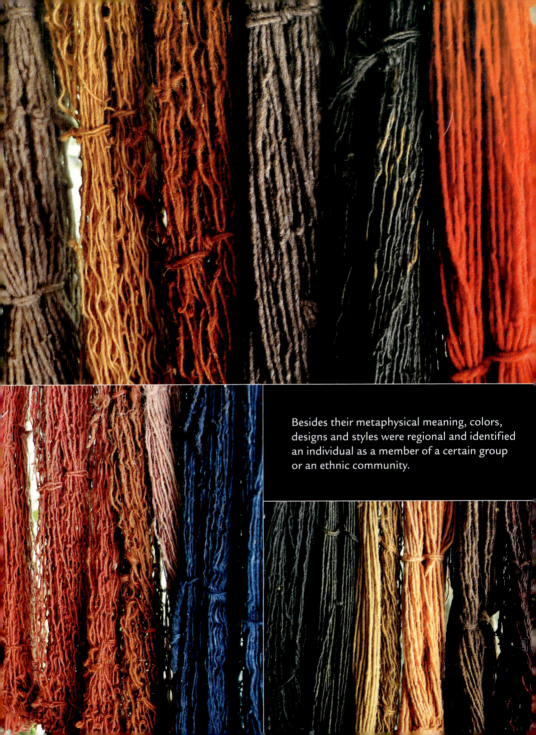

Besides their metaphysical meaning, colors, designs and styles were regional and identified an individual as a member of a certain group or an ethnic community.

# Fire Bush

## Spanish Name: Sanalotodo
### Scientific Name: Hamelia patens Jacq.

In traditional medicine the leaves of fire bush are used for all kinds of skin conditions, sores, rashes, wounds, burns, itching, cuts, skin fungus, insect stings and bites. Fresh leaves may be added to homemade anti-septic herbal salves.

Local farmers chewed on a leaf of fire bush while working in the heat because of its cooling qualities.

Dried and powdered leaves were traditionally applied in case of infected umbilical cord.

Toasted leaves are applied on boils.

To calm itching from bites, hives and to alleviate rheumatism a gallon of water in which 2 handfuls of fire bush leaves have been boiled is used as a rinse.

For wasp or bee stings the juice from a heated leaf is applied directly to the affected area.

Fire bush is a tall fast growing plant seen in sunny places throughout the Yucatan. In the Mayan language it is called *Ix-Canan* which means "the guardian of the forest". In the Spanish language it is called *sanalotodo* which translates as "cure all" because of its many medicinal properties.

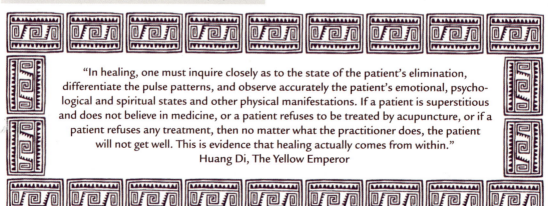

"In healing, one must inquire closely as to the state of the patient's elimination, differentiate the pulse patterns, and observe accurately the patient's emotional, psychological and spiritual states and other physical manifestations. If a patient is superstitious and does not believe in medicine, or a patient refuses to be treated by acupuncture, or if a patient refuses any treatment, then no matter what the practitioner does, the patient will not get well. This is evidence that healing actually comes from within."
Huang Di, The Yellow Emperor

# roadside plants

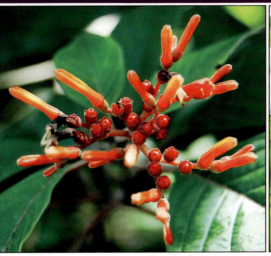
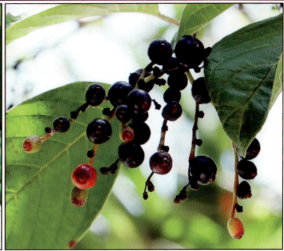

The small bright flowers are edible before they turn into black berries.

## Natural Clay

Clay was used all around the world as a medicinal or a cosmetic remedy for many centuries. It comes in a great variety: red, green, white, grey, and can range from very fine to quite coarse.

Below: White cosmetic clay draws out impurities without removing the natural oils, while exfoliating, cleansing and stimulating the circulation. This white clay from a local cenote is suitable for all types of skin.

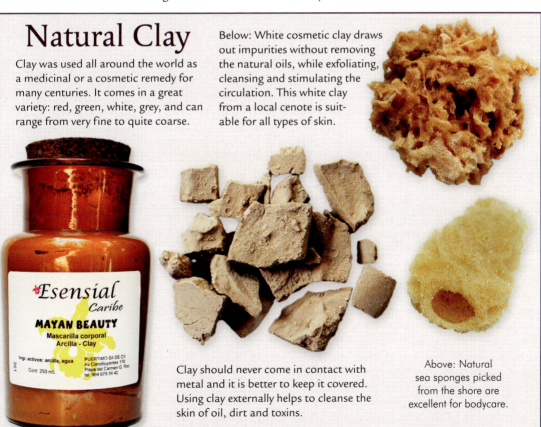

Clay should never come in contact with metal and it is better to keep it covered. Using clay externally helps to cleanse the skin of oil, dirt and toxins.

Above: Natural sea sponges picked from the shore are excellent for bodycare.

# Mayan Clay

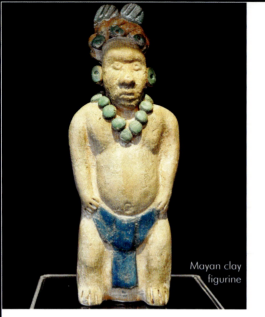

Mayan clay figurine

Clay is a true and rare gift of the earth; for many thousands of years it provided shelter, holding vessels, medicine, dyes, and material upon which history was recorded and is ever present in the mythology of many civilizations. Clay may have been one of the first materials used by humans: the heat of the sun was sufficient to keep it in shape, and the heat of the fire shaped it forever.

The Mayan civilization is well known for its fine clay and stonework, and the Yucatan Peninsula was a place famous for its figurines, round jars, cylindrical vases, shallow flat bottomed plates, tripod jars and decorated incense burners.

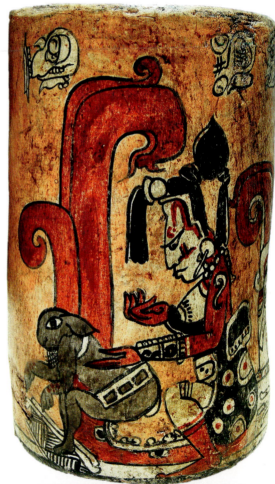

The ancient Maya molded or hand shaped their clay as the potter's wheel was never invented in Mesoamerica. A very recent discovery revealed that the Mayan blue color, used for masks, sculptures, codices, decorations, fresco painting and household pottery was also made of clay, the scientific name of which is *palygorkite,* deposits of which were found in Uxmal, Ticul and a few other places. It was made by combining clay with the indigo color, extracted from the plant with the same name. The Mayan blue proved to be extremely resistant to time and damage. It was, in fact, a precursor to modern high-tech hybrids that often combine organic and non-organic materials.

In the Mayan communities of the present, clay pots and bowls are still used for cooking and the raw materials are usually found nearby the potter's home. Tical remains a place which kept its pottery traditions for many centuries and the finest replicas that are exhibited in the anthropological museums of many cities come from there. White clay from the Caribbean coast and yellow from the mountain area of Chiapas are well appreciated as part of folk medicine and a remedy for rashes, mumps, stomach problems and insect and snake bites.

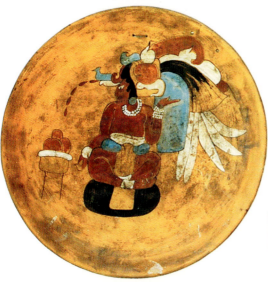

Clay is a unique material because its particles are very small. They are so small that they can carry an electric charge, a negative one, therefore internally clay is believed to be able to attract and cleanse the digestive tract of positively charged ions, which promote the growth of bacteria, fungi and parasites.

Clay is also a natural source of many trace minerals, including calcium, magnesium and zinc, all of which are beneficial for the skin, relieve pain and revitalize the body.

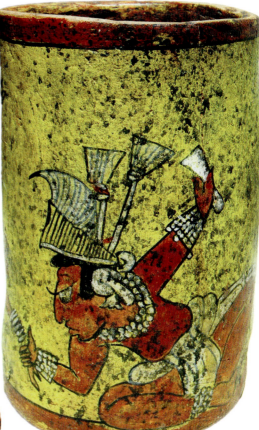

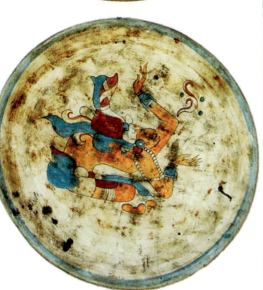

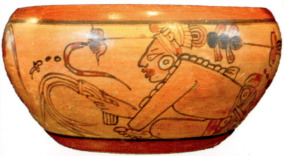

The museum quality replicas of ancient Mayan pottery shown on these pages are made by contemporary artists using the same materials and techniques as in antiquity. Many of the pottery workshops are located around Ticul.

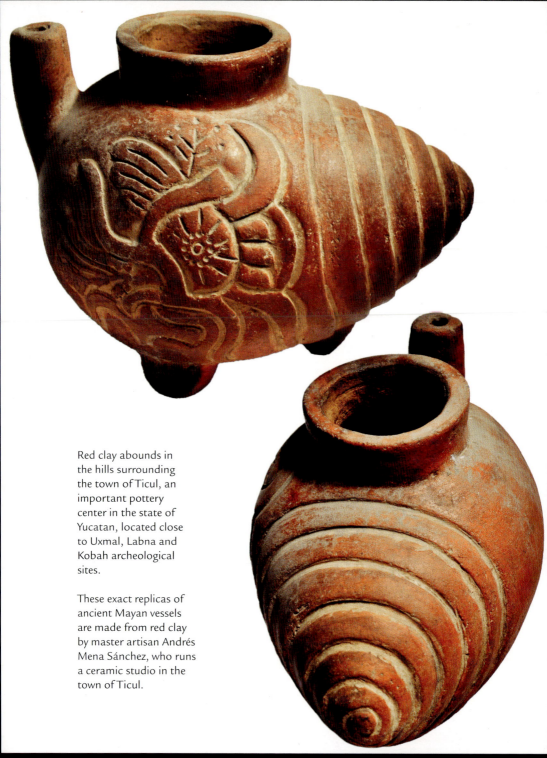

Red clay abounds in the hills surrounding the town of Ticul, an important pottery center in the state of Yucatan, located close to Uxmal, Labna and Kobah archeological sites.

These exact replicas of ancient Mayan vessels are made from red clay by master artisan Andrés Mena Sánchez, who runs a ceramic studio in the town of Ticul.

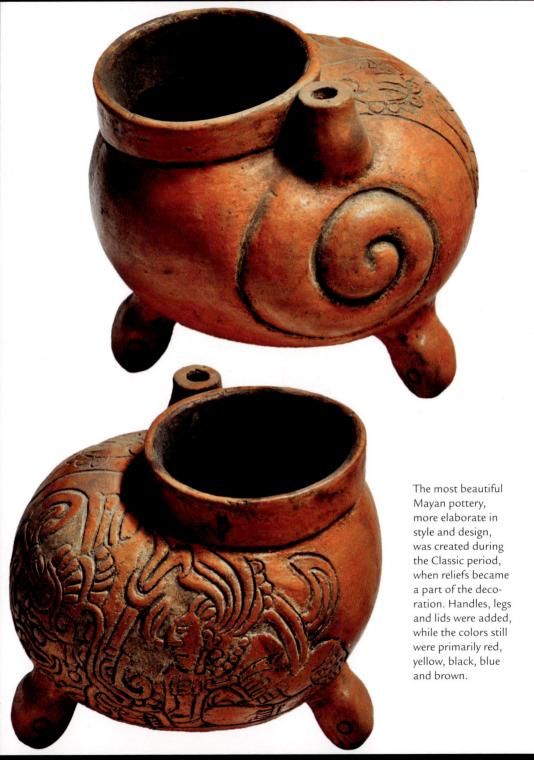

The most beautiful Mayan pottery, more elaborate in style and design, was created during the Classic period, when reliefs became a part of the decoration. Handles, legs and lids were added, while the colors still were primarily red, yellow, black, blue and brown.

# Flamboyant

### Spanish Name: Tabachín
### Scientific Name: Caesalpinia pulcherrima L.

For sad or depressed people a handful of leaves and flowers is added to 4 l of cold water and the mix is placed in the sunlight for the entire day. After sunset the liquid is filtered and used as a rinse after a shower or a bath. This procedure is more effective if repeated for 3 consecutive days.

A decoction made with fresh leaves was traditionally used as a liver tonic.

An infusion made with bark, leaves and roots was used for a variety of conditions ranging from colds and fevers to skin diseases.

A decoction of boiled leaves clears mouth and throat ulcers. **It cannot be swallowed!**

A decoction made of fresh flowers was used as a rinse for minor eye inflammations.

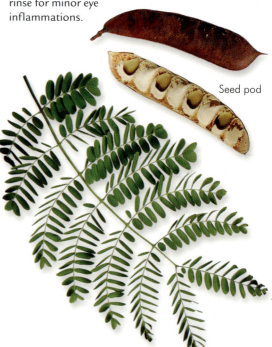
Seed pod

A small evergreen tree from the West Indies, flamboyant usually does not grow taller than 3-5 m. The stems and branches have spines and it is very common in the forests and towns of the Yucatan Peninsula. It is also called peacock flower, or red/yellow bird of paradise. The flowers of this plant are used locally in traditional rituals and ceremonies.

"The function and duty of a quality human being is a sincere and honest development of one's potential."
Bruce Lee
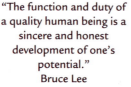

# roadside plants

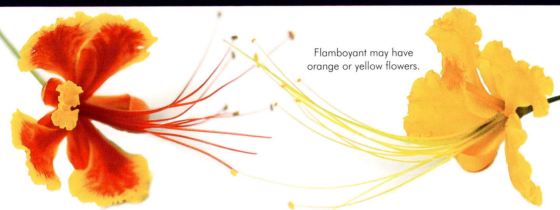

Flamboyant may have orange or yellow flowers.

# Basket & Mat Making

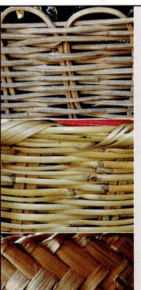

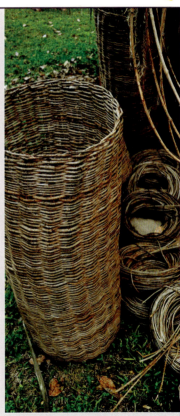

Basketry and matting were an important part of Mesoamerican commercial activity. Many different plants were used for fibers of which the most common throughout the Mayan world were palm trees, sugar cane, *sisal, henequen,* bamboo, vines, tree branches and specially prepared cuttings of wood. Harvesting plant fibers was done in accordance with the Moon cycles to ensure their durability and to keep them free of insects.

The use of baskets in antiquity by the Maya is depicted on the stelae at the archeological sites of Yaxchilan and Oxkhintok.

The *petate* is a thin woven mat, called *pop* in most Mayan languages, most often made of the leaves of palm of petate *(Leucothrinax morrisii)*. Mayan codices show people sitting on mats or placing offerings to the deities on mats. The statues of the Mayan gods were also always placed on a mat.

The *petate* was used for sleeping and rolled up to hang during the day. Seeds, nuts, corn and *tortillas* were dried in the sun on a mat.

A basket is called a *canasta* if it has handles, or *canasto* if it does not.

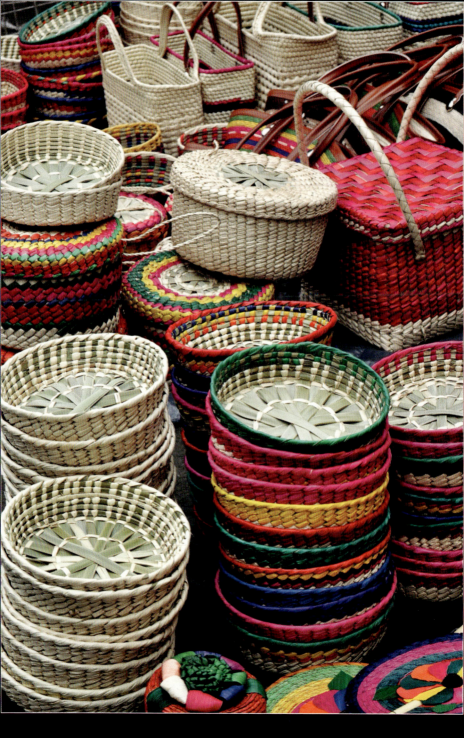

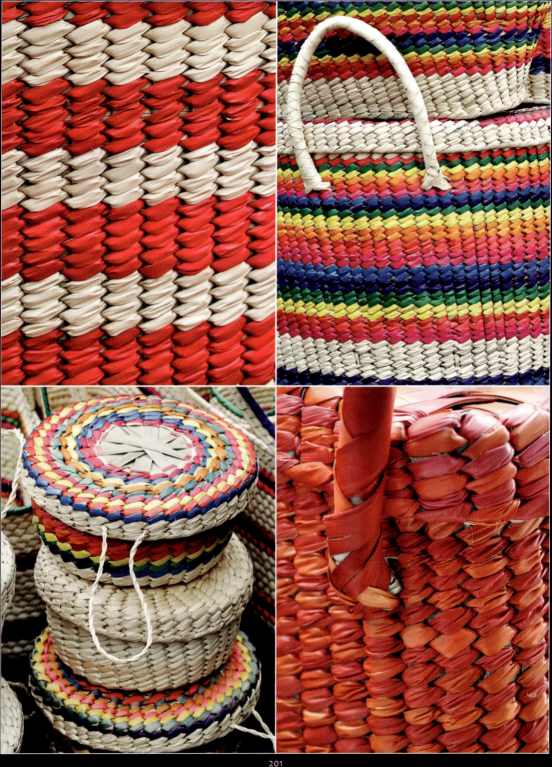

# Gumbolimbo Tree

## Spanish Name: Chaka
### Scientific Name: Bursera simaruba

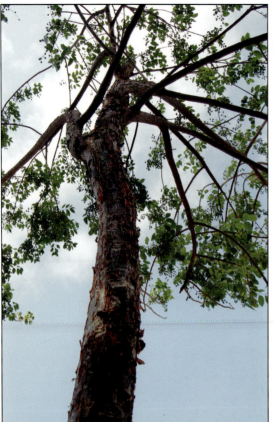

The *chaka* is the antidote for the poisonous sap of the *chechen* tree. If the sap from the chechen tree gets anywhere on the body one must cut off a piece of *chaka* bark and quickly apply it on the affected area. A rinse can be made by putting finely chopped bark into the water and letting it stand for a couple of hours.

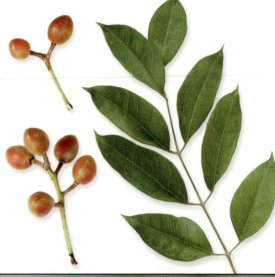

*Chaka* is a large tree abundant in the Yucatan. It is easy to recognize because of its brown peeling bark. It is interesting that *chaka* and *chechen* very often grow close to each other. If the bark is cut off the tree it has to be done in vertical stripes. The bark can never be cut out as a ring around the trunk because it injures the tree permanently.

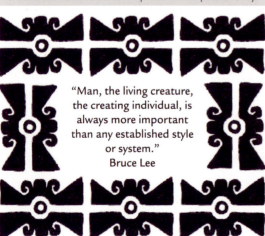

"Man, the living creature, the creating individual, is always more important than any established style or system."
Bruce Lee

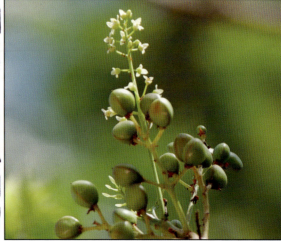

# roadside plants

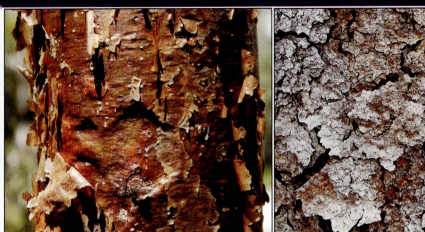

The gumbalino tree is easy to identify because of its bright brown peeling bark.

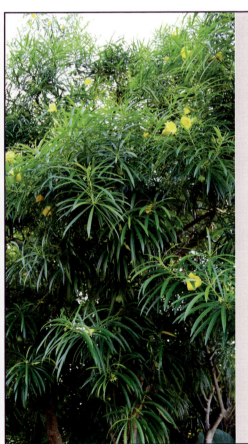

## Ayoyote
### Thevetia gaumery

*Ayoyote* originated in the West Indies and is an evergreen tropical tree that is usually 5-8 m tall. It is very common throughout Central America. The flowers may be yellow or light orange. It is very pleasant looking and is used frequently as an ornamental tree.

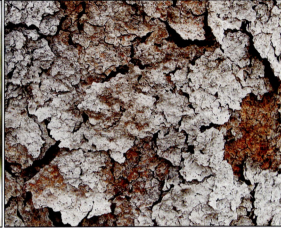

The sap, fruit and seeds are poisonous and cannot be eaten

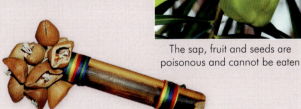

Dried and cut nuts from different trees are used in rituals and ceremonies. Sometimes they are made to be worn by dancers on their wrists or ankles to make a rattling sound. They are also used in other indigenous musical instruments.

# Hibiscus

**SPANISH NAME: TULIPÁN**
**SCIENTIFIC NAME: HIBISCUS ROSA-SINENSIS L.**

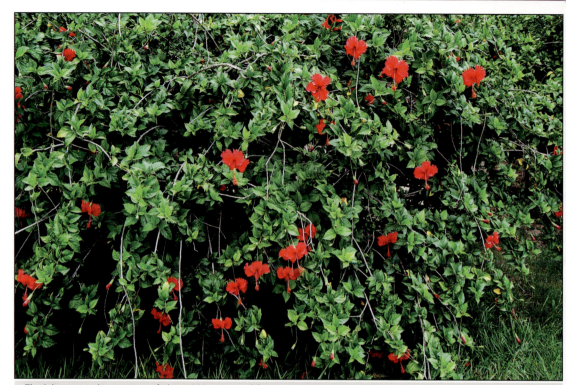

The hibiscus is a large genus of about 250 species of flowering plants in the *Malvaceae* family now common to temperate, tropical and subtropical climate zones. Hibiscus has been cultivated for so long that there are no records of the wild flower it originated from. One species of Hibiscus known as *Kenaf (Hibiscus Cannabinus)* is extensively used in paper making. Another, *Roselle (Hibiscus Sabdariffa)* is used as a vegetable and to make herbal teas and jams, especially in the Caribbean. Dry petals of its flower are sold as jamaica. In Mexico the jamaica drink is extremely popular and is made at home and commercially.

Red hibiscus flowers may be used medicinally. Select the flowers grown in environmentally clean areas. They are edible and very rich in iron. For anemia eat 1-2 flowers. Flower extract is a remedy for liver disorders and high blood pressure.

Minor skin problems may be helped if an infusion of leaves and flowers is added to a bath.

Local midwives use a decoction made with 9 leaves and 2 flowers (1 open and 1 closed) in 3 glasses of water boiled for 10 minutes to reduce postpartum bleeding.

For headaches and fever mashed leaves are applied as a poultice directly on the forehead.

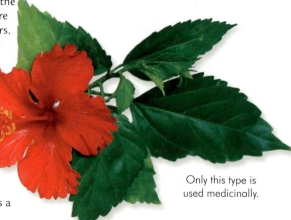

Only this type is used medicinally.

# roadside plants

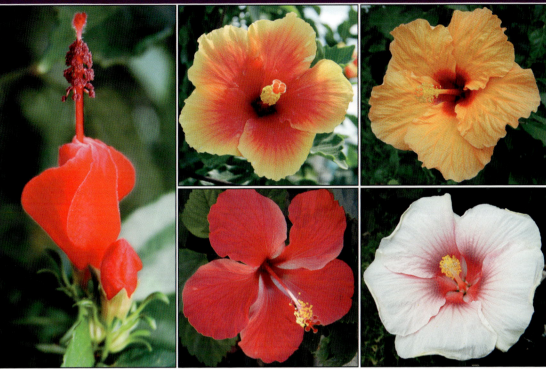

Above left: A wild variety, *Malvaviscus arboreus*

Above right: The decorative varieties cannot be used medicinally.

# Ponche - a Mexican winter beverage

Jamaica- dried hibiscus flower (*Hibiscus sabdariffa L.*)

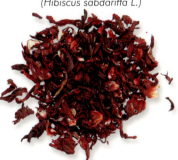

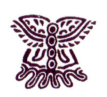
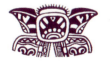

200 g of brown cane sugar

150 g of tamarind

2-3 liters of water

200 g of prunes

300 g of *guayava*

50 g of jamaica

300 g of *tejocote*

2-4 sticks of cinnamon

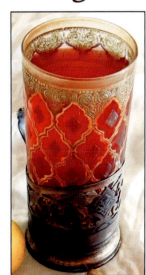

Cook all ingredients in a 4 liter pot on a low fire for 40-50 minutes. Serve warm or chilled; honey and lime is optional.

# Orchid

## SPANISH NAME: ORQUIDEA
### SCIENTIFIC NAME: ORCHIDACEAE

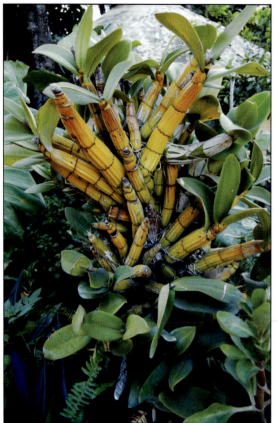

Along with the decorative use of the flowers, over 50 species of orchid plants are used in traditional Chinese medicine. Most often the stems, bulbs or roots are sold dried. In tropical countries plants can also be found fresh at herbal markets.

Some orchid flowers are made into tea, a very fine and rare beverage.

Some species have been used for immune system support, others for different types of nervous conditions, intestinal parasites and tropical fevers.

Some varieties are prepared into ointments for skin infections and poultices.

Ointment made of *Aplestrum hyemale* is used as a remedy for underskin abscesses. The leaves of *Vanda hootieriana* are used as a warm compress for arthritis pain.

In antiquity this plant was used as an aphrodisiac.

Fresh bulb (right) cut in half and toasted was later applied externally upon bruises and minor injuries.

Orchids are biologically complex plants, prized for their beautiful flowers with very pleasant and fine fragrances. There are over twenty thousand wild species and seventy thousand hybrids, making the orchid one of the most diverse plants in existence. In natural environments orchids are most often found as bulbs that grow on old trees or rocks and survive with very little moisture for extended periods of time. This adaptation allows orchid plant to accumulate a lot of nutrients and organic substances that nourish the plant during dry heat. Orchids are common in Central America and almost any tall tree has some growing on it. They survive very well in parks and other eco-friendly manmade environments. The presence of orchids in the forest is one of the indicators of its health. The name of the plant comes from the Greek word *"orchis"*.

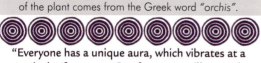

"Everyone has a unique aura, which vibrates at a particular frequency. Our frequency will not only determine who and what we like or dislike, but also what experiences and people we attract in life."
Alchemy of Love Relationships, Joseph Michael Levry

Orchid bulb

Dried orchid bulb

Seed pod

# roadside plants

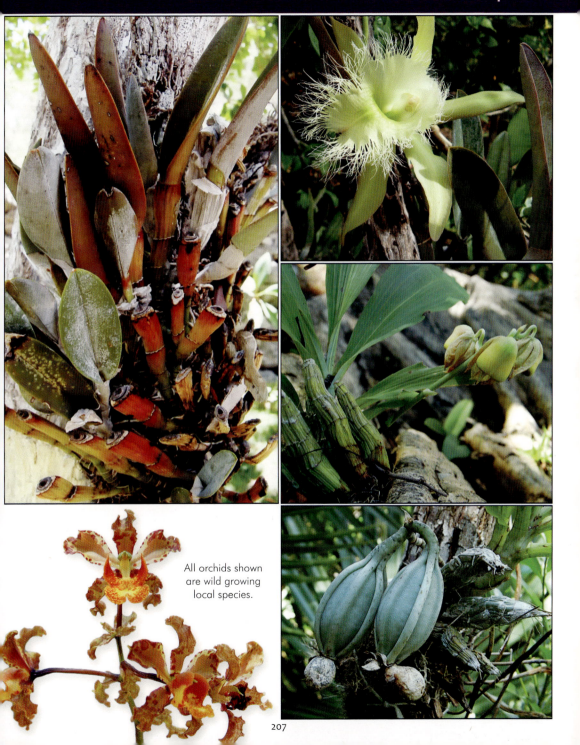

All orchids shown are wild growing local species.

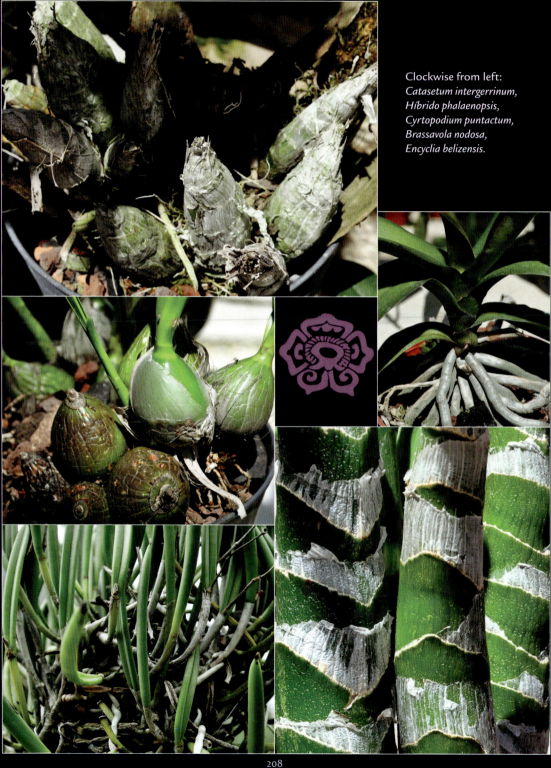

Clockwise from left:
*Catasetum intergerrinum,*
*Híbrido phalaenopsis,*
*Cyrtopodium puntactum,*
*Brassavola nodosa,*
*Encyclia belizensis.*

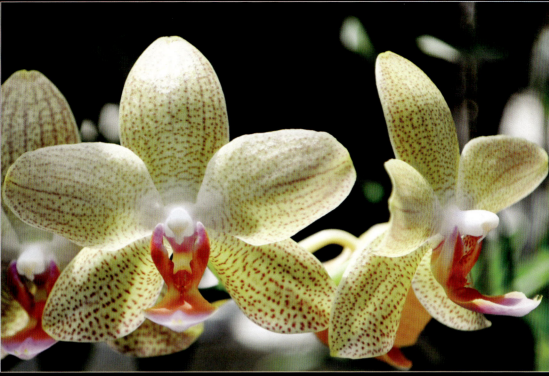
The orchid pavilion in Xcaret exhibits species native to the Mexican Caribbean, many of which are endangered.

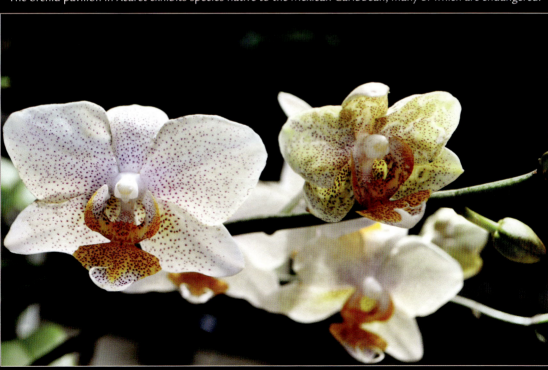

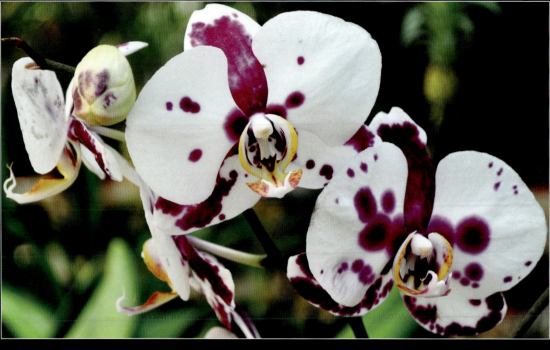

"Keep your love of nature, for that is the true way to understand art more and more."
Vincent van Gogh

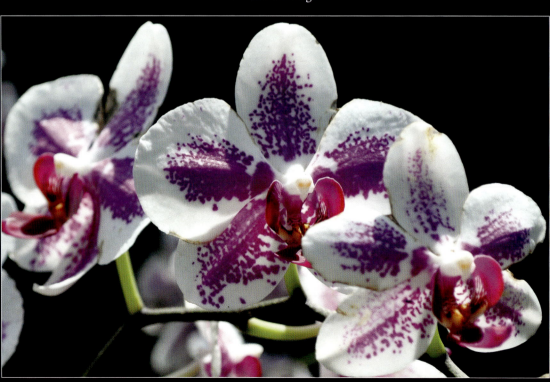

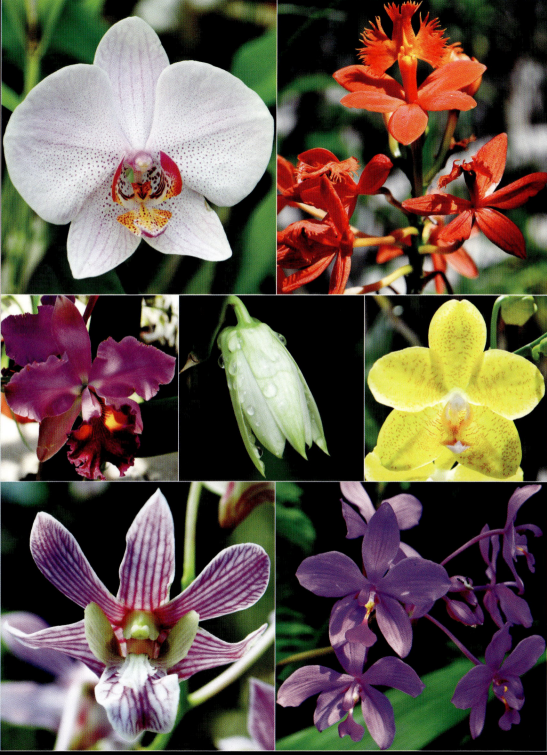

# Vanilla
## Vainilla
### Vanilla planifolio

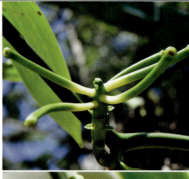

Vanilla is a flavoring that is derived from the orchid *Vanilla Planifolio,* native to Mexico, that was cultivated by the ancient inhabitants of Mesoamerica and well appreciated by the Aztecs. It was introduced to Europe in the XVI century, but all the attempts to cultivate vanilla orchids outside of Mexico were failing for almost 300 years, because these orchids depend on tiny *Melipona* bees which pollinate them. In the middle of the XIX century hand pollination of vanilla orchids was discovered and vanilla cultivation quickly spread to other tropical regions.

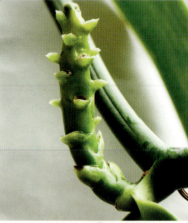

At present time there are three kinds of vanilla orchids that are grown commercially: *Vanilla tahitensis, Vanilla Pompon* and the most common, *Vanilla planifolio.* Growing vanilla orchids requires a lot of work, making it one of the most expensive spices in the world. It is used in cooking, baking, aromatherapy, and with drinks such as coffee and chocolate. If tiny vanilla seeds appear as dark specks in a flavored dish it indicates that whole natural vanilla beans were used to prepare it. Medicinally vanilla has been used as an aphrodisiac, to reduce fever and calm the nerves and stomach.

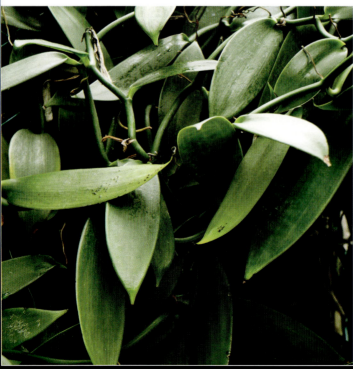

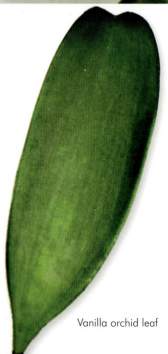

Vanilla orchid leaf

The vanilla orchid is a vine that needs the support of another plant in order to grow. The top part of the plant is folded down to stimulate the plant to produce more flowers. A pollinated flower produces one fruit – a deep green bean pod with tiny black seeds. *Vanilla planifolia* flowers are hermaphroditic: they carry both anther and the stigma, separated by a membrane to prevent self-pollination. A vanilla flower lasts only one day, and if not pollinated, it loses its chance to make a fruit.

The fruit is a seed capsule which may ripen on a plant, turning black and slightly dusty in appearance, then releasing the distinctive smell; or they can be harvested when green but fully mature.

It is easier to grow vanilla orchids from the cuttings of older plants than starting them from the seeds, which require the presence of a certain fungi in order to germinate. A part of the vine with 7-10 leaves is cut and planted close to the parent plant, where it may grow very rapidly if the conditions are beneficial.

Natural vanilla extract is easy to prepare at home by cutting ripe vanilla beans into small pieces and placing them into vodka or tequila for a few weeks.

Tonka bean extract, sometimes sold as vanilla or added to commercial vanilla extract, may be harmful for people's health.

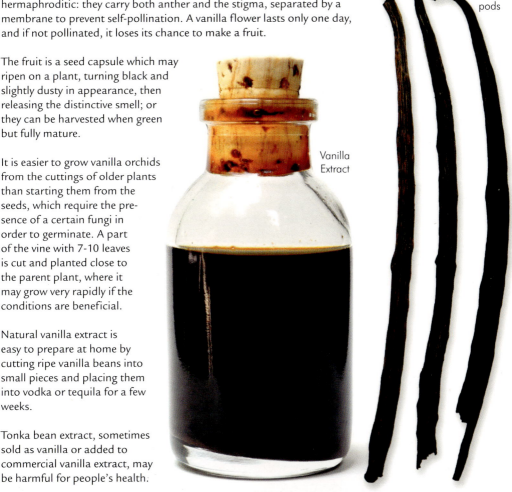

Vanilla Extract

Dried pods

# Coffee
## Árbol de Café
### Coffea

Coffee plants are shrubs or small trees usually reaching the height of 3-4 m. Several varietes are grown for beans made into a drink. The coffee plant, native to Africa, was brought to Mexico in the end of the XVII century.

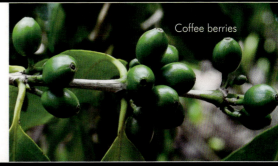

Coffee berries

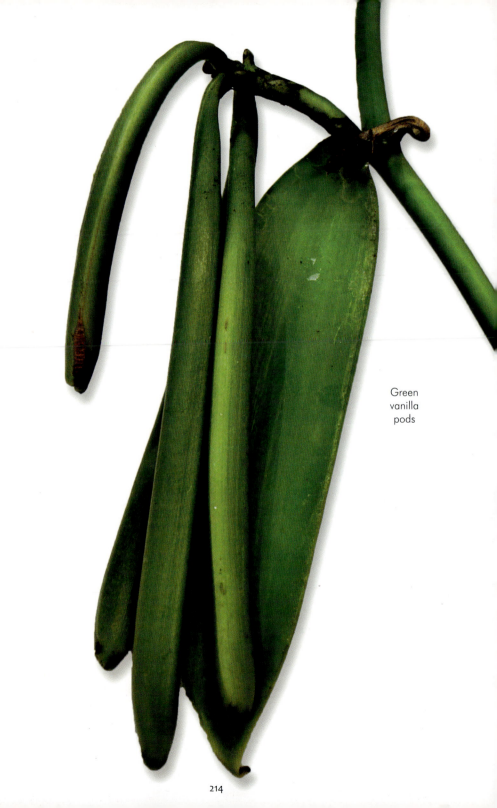

Green vanilla pods

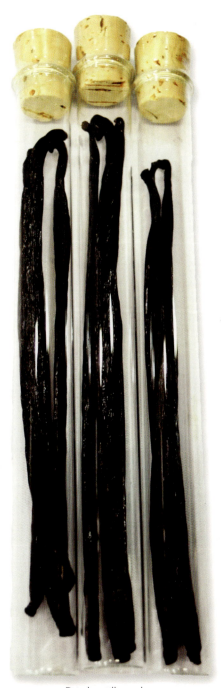

Dried vanilla pods

# Passionfruit

## Spanish Name: Marakuya
### Scientific Name: Passiflora edulis

Passionfruit as a plant is one of the best remedies for all types of nervous conditions; it has a calming and relaxing effect on the entire organism, stimulates good sleep, relieves muscular tension, lowers blood pressure and soothes pain. The infusion is prepared with 6-7 g of dry leaves for 150 ml of water and taken 3 times a day after meals.

Passionfruit leaves in infusions are a good remedy for irritability and insomnia that does not create an addiction. This infusion is recommended for muscular spasms resulted from asthma and intestinal disorders of nervous origins.

Syrup made with honey is a preventative remedy for seizures and hysteria.

For laryngitis the infusion of 5 g of leaves in 500 ml of water is taken 3 times a day after meals.

Passionfruit is very beneficial for the heart, stomach ulcers, kidneys and it regulates blood pressure.

Passionfruit is a very common vine in the tropical Americas from a family with over 500 different species. The most common in the Mexican Caribbean are *Passiflorae incaranata*, *Passiflorae alba*, and *Passiflorae yucatenesis*. The vine gently attaches to other trees without harming them. Passionfruit is a fruit from one variety of *Passiflora* harvested in the wild and available in fruit markets.

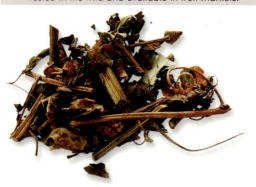

The aerial parts of the plant are used in dry or fresh form prepared into an infusion or a tincture.

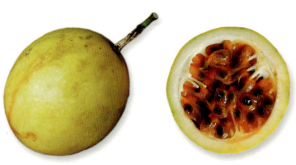

*Marakuya* fruit is prized for its delicious flavor

# roadside plants

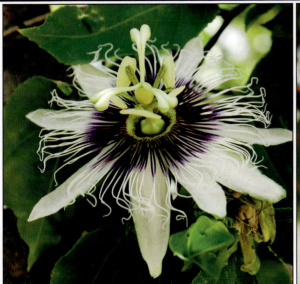

Passionfruit flowers open for just one day and have a strong, delightfully pleasant fragrance.

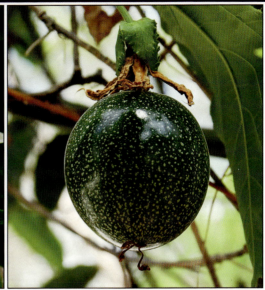

It is important to consume *marakuya* fruit when well ripened; when green it is toxic.

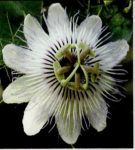

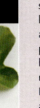

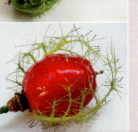

## Passion Flower
### Pasiflora

This is one of many varieties of the same family. The flowers and leaves are much smaller, while the fruit is only about 2 cm long. The delicate hairs that hold the fruit are very fragrant. Leaves and flowers prepared in a decoction of 20 g of herb for 1 l of water are used externally to clear minor skin inflammations. Passionflower infusion has sedative and anti-spasmodic qualities.

Both *marakuya* and pasiflora can be propagated from the seeds and it is best to plant them in the spring.

They like medium shadow areas and need the support of another tree or plant.

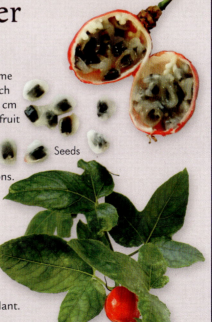

Seeds

# Periwinkle

## Spanish Name: Vicaria
### Scientific Name: Catharanthus roseus L.

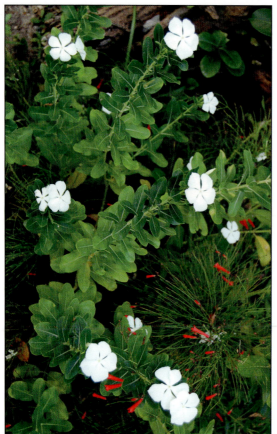

Periwinkle is thought to have originated in Madagascar and spread to all the tropics. It is a small plant, 50-80 cm tall, easily recognizable because of its bright flowers, white or pink, and it is very abundant everywhere in the Yucatan. In herbal medicine fresh flowers, leaves and roots are used. Other decorative varieties that come in many different colors cannot be used medicinally.

The flowers of white periwinkle were used in an eye rinse or eye drops for tired eyes. In 1 glass of water 8 flowers are made in an infusion, cooled off, and one drop is taken in the morning and one drop at night.

Only the pink periwinkle has alkaloids that in studies detained the growth of tumors.

The aerial parts of pink periwinkle have properties that regulate high blood pressure and are beneficial for people with diabetes. The same decoction is believed to alleviate some discomfort associated with menopause.

For sore throat pink flowers in an infusion may be used as a gargle.

Only the two varieties shown here are used medicinally.

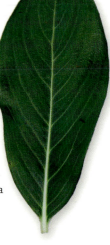

"Herbs have many properties that modern science has yet to discover. Herbs are forgotten foods because they have been eliminated from our diets through the process of selection which, over the course of thousands of years, has rejected foods that were unappealing to eyes, nose or mouth, and as man learned to cultivate his own food, he naturally chose to cultivate only those foods that appealed to his senses. As the saying goes, we are what we eat. If we eat stronger foods, we become stronger ourselves. If we eat better foods, our health improves. Herbs give everlasting strength while regular foods give only temporary strength."
Dr. Stephen T. Chang, The Tao of Sexology, The Book of Infinite Wisdom

# roadside plants

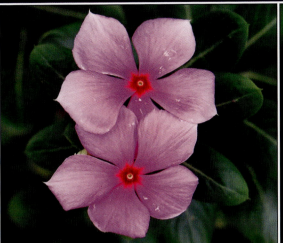
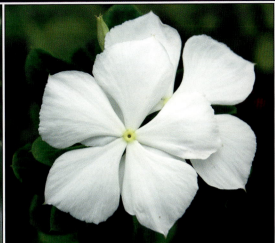

Only the pink and white varieties of periwinkle are used medicinally.

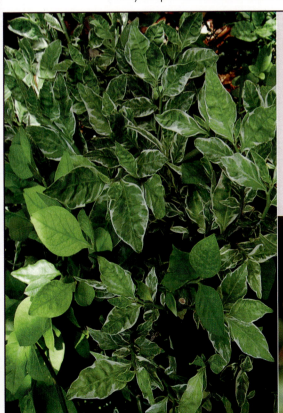

# Bienvenida
## Pedilanthus tithymaloides

*Bienvenida* is a small shrub that grows 1-2 m high and is used ornamentally. Traditionally it has been planted by the Maya close to the entrance of the house in order to bring prosperity and welcome benevolent spirits.

A branch 20 to 30 cm long can be cut off and planted immediately. It likes sun and moisture.

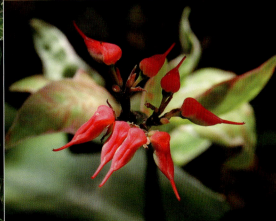

Spanish Name: Uva del Mar
Scientific Name: Coccoloba uvifera L.

# Seagrapes

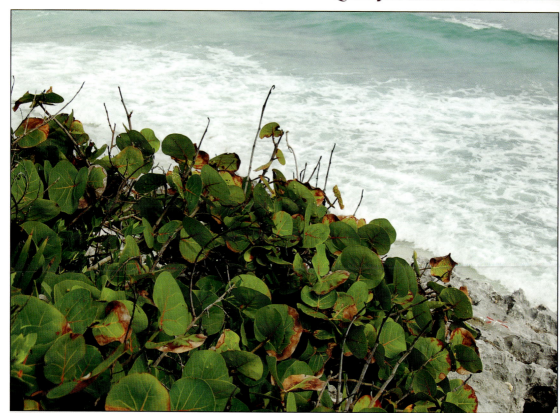

Seagrapes is a tree that can grow quite tall and is native to the sandy shores of the tropical Americas. This plant is very resistant to damage from the elements and is commonly used for decoration of seaside gardens. The small fruit resembles grapes, with 40-50 on a single cluster. They are edible raw or can be made into a marmelade. The pulp of the fruit is of a pleasant sweet and sour taste and has a small seed.

Leaves in an infusion have a soothing effect on the vocal cords, and may be used as an anti-septic rinse.

The bark of the tree is astringent and was used as a tonic for chronic digestive infections.

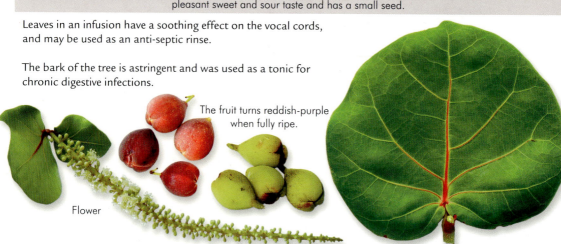

The fruit turns reddish-purple when fully ripe.

Flower

# roadside plants

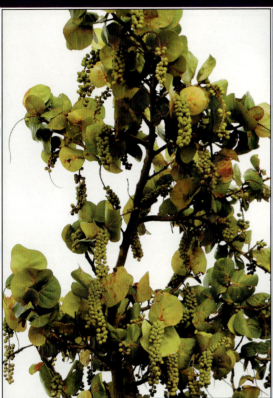
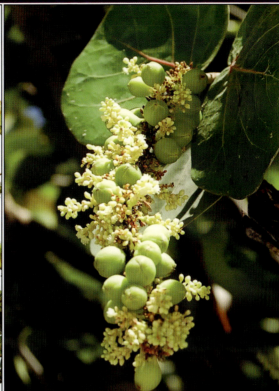

## Railroad Vine
### Riñonina
#### Ipomoea pes-caprae

Railroad vine is a fast growing beach plant. It can be recognized by its bright pink flowers.

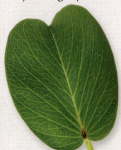

A decoction made from the plant is used to treat mild kidney disorders.

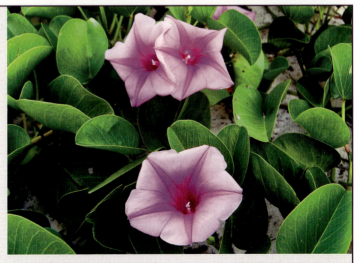

A poultice of the leaves mixed with the liquid from the boiled root are used on abscesses and to reduce swelling.

**Spanish Name: Aceitilla**
Scientific Name: Bidens pilosa L.

# Spanish Needle

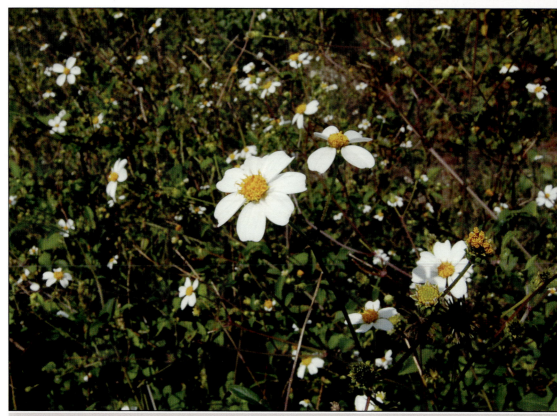

*Aceitilla* is native to the Western Hemisphere and is a perennial herb from the same family as feverfew, usually not more than 1 m tall. It can grow even in very poor and rocky soil along roads, trails and open lowland areas and thrives in sunny spots. It spreads very easily, attaching its seeds to human clothing, birds and animals. For medicinal purposes the entire plant may be used. It is very common in the Yucatan Peninsula.

*Acetilla* is traditionally used in infusions to reduce inflammation related to minor infections and to lower blood sugar, thus being a good herb for diabetes.

In a decoction it may be used as a tonic for the urinary and reproductive systems, to promote menstruation, stimulate liver function and expel worms.

The entire plant is used externally for kidney or liver inflammation when uprooted and prepared into a poultice.

Ointment made with flowers and leaves is rich in estrogen and when applied and massaged gently on the lower abdomen it is a remedy for menopause.

A drop of juice from a fresh plant on a piece of cotton is helpful for earache.

Tea made with acetilla is beneficial for hypertension or as a mouth rinse for ulcers.

**High doses can irritate kidneys.**

Seed pod

# roadside plants

# Wild Balsam Apple
## Sorosi
### Momordica charantia L.

Wild balsam apple is a vine from the family of *cucurbitáceas* that grows wild in dry and sunny spots. It is a relative of the balsam apple, which has similar leaves and fruit 10-15 cm long, edible when still green. Wild balsam apple has a very small fruit, 5 cm in length with red, sticky seeds inside.

Wild balsam apple leaves are used in infusions for intestinal colic, slow digestion, parasites and as a liver tonic.

The red pulp from the seeds is used externally in the preparation of ointments for abscesses and tumors.

For some skin conditions a decoction of the aerial parts is used as a rinse: 60 g of fresh herb for 1 l of water is boiled for 30 minutes on low heat.
The same decoction added to bath water is used as an insecticide against ticks and lice.

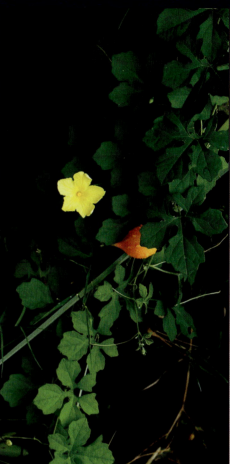

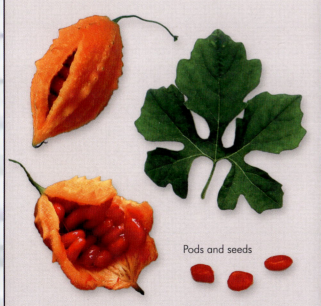

Pods and seeds

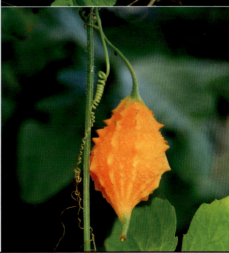

# Thornapple
## Toloache
### Datura Innoxia

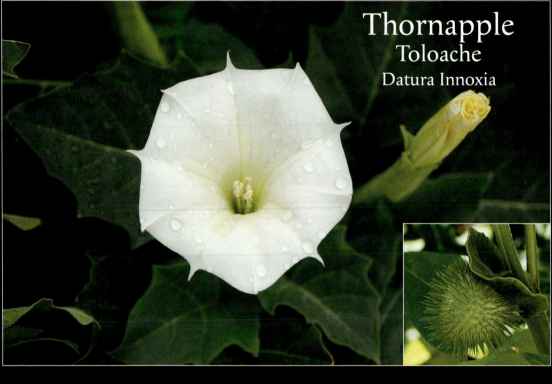

Thornapple is a shrub growing to 2 m in height in sunny spots with little moisture. It is native to the American continent. In the Yucatan these plants are called *toloache* and are used only by very experienced herbalists. *All parts of this plant are toxic and accidental consumption of even a single leaf may lead to severe effects.* Medicinally aerial parts of the plant are used for external application for rheumatic pain, varicose veins, arthritis, skin inflammations and wounds.

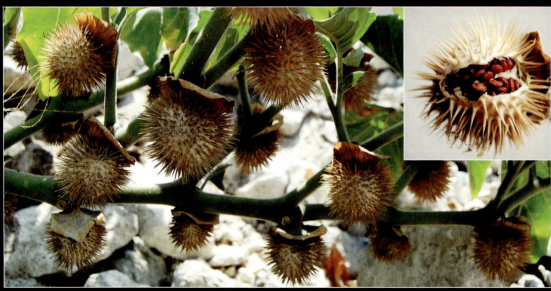

# Datura Metel

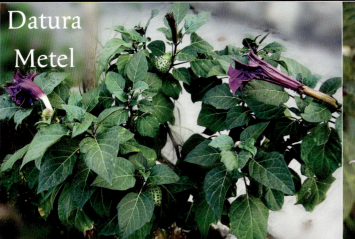
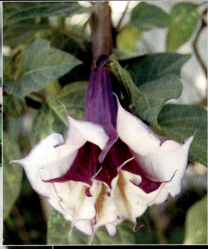

Datura Arborea or *Brugmansia Arborea* is characterized by big white flowers that earned it the name Angel's Trumpet. In South America parts of the plants are taken in infusion or smoked in order to produce visions.

Medicinally it is used by local healers for tetanus or as an anesthetic (below left & right).

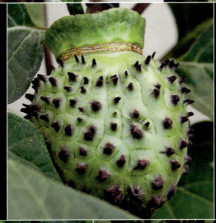

*Datura Metel* is a close relative of *Datura Inoxia*. It is a stunningly beautiful plant, with big flowers that may reach 10 cm in length. Colors range from white to creamy yellow, orange, red and purple. The flowers may be single or double. *Datura Metel* is one of the fundamental 50 herbs used in Chinese herbology (above).

## Brugmansia Arborea

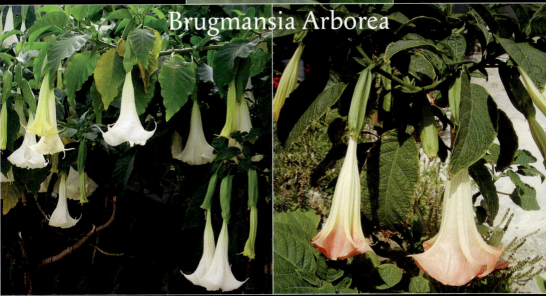

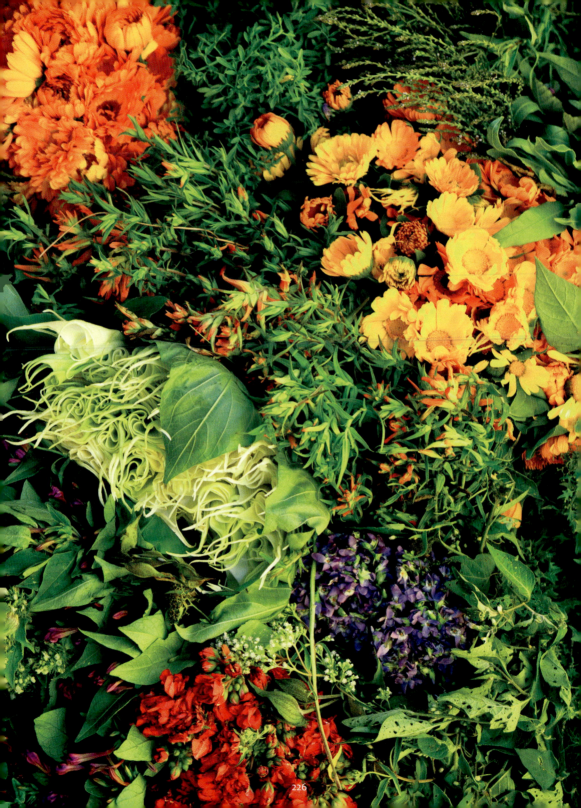

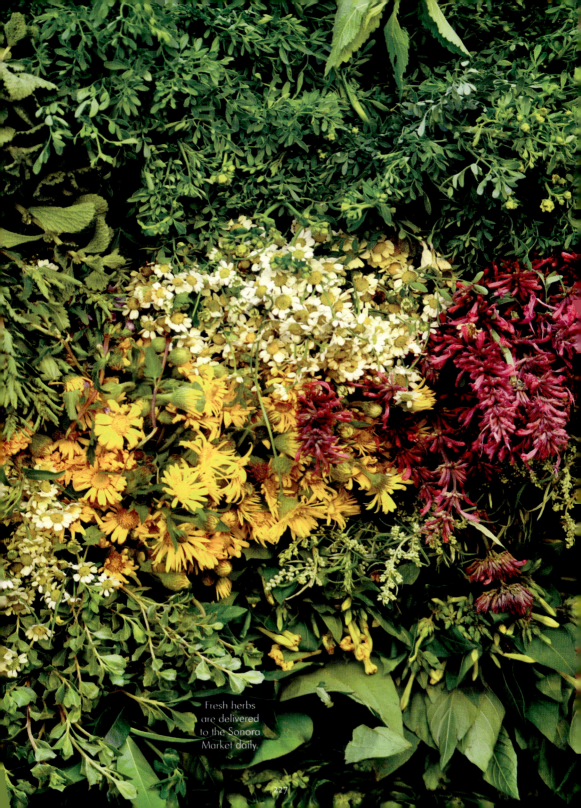

Fresh herbs are delivered to the Sonora Market daily.

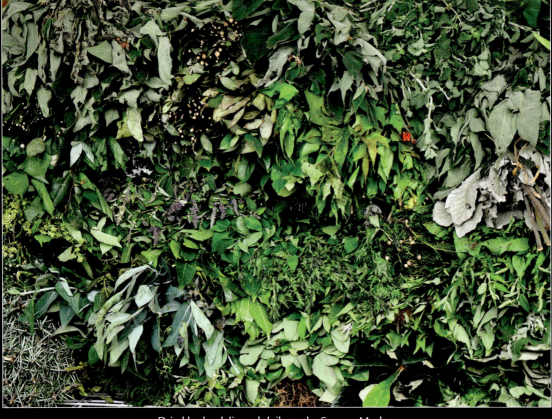
Dried herbs delivered daily to the Sonora Market.

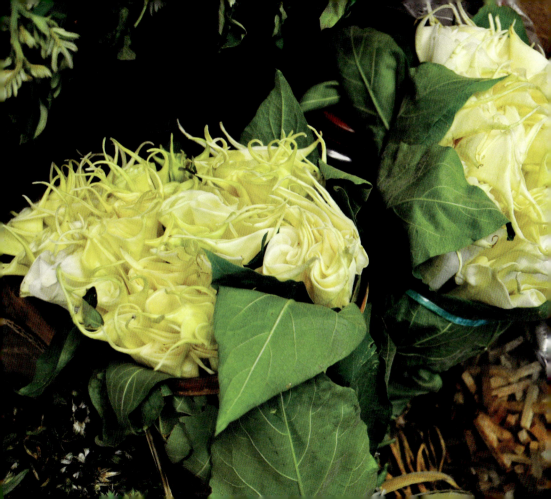

# Water Lily

**SPANISH NAME: NINFEA**
**SCIENTIFIC NAME: NYMPHAEA ODORATA**

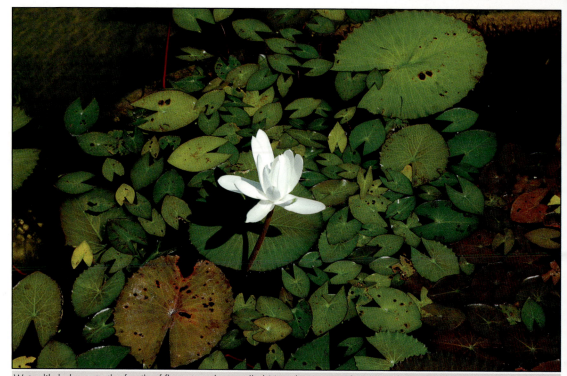

Water lily belongs to the family of flowering plants called *Nymphaeaceae*. There are about 70 different species around the world that live in fresh water in temperate and tropical climates. The tropical water lilies flower during the day and night, while the hardy variety only opens flowers during the day. It is very abundant in the Yucatan Peninsula in cenotes and lagoons because it grows very well in slow moving water.

The medicinal qualities of the white lily *(Nymphaea Odorata)* were very well known to the native people of the Americas. The dried root has astringent and mucilaginous properties. It was usually harvested in the autumn, cleaned of mud, sliced and dried. When dried it can be used to make alcohol tincture (25% root, 75% alcohol) or can be powdered and macerated in boiling water for some time to prepare an infusion.

Tincture or infusion was used to treat gastro-intestinal and respiratory conditions.

Leaves and dried roots in a poultice are considered a good external remedy for skin lesions and inflammations related to mucous membranes. In traditional medicine and infusion and internal rinse was used for cancer of the uterus and other less severe disorders.

> "Intuition is the guidance of the soul. It is the soul talking to us guiding us through the jungle of life. A person without intuition or inner hearing has neither direction nor command."
> Lifting the Veil, Joseph Michael Levry

# roadside plants

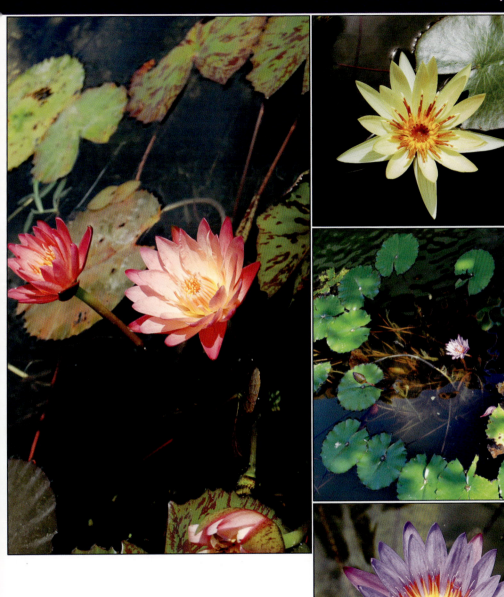

The beauty of the water lily led to its widespread ornamental use. In the Spanish language the flower is sometimes called *ninfa de las aguas,* or water nymph.

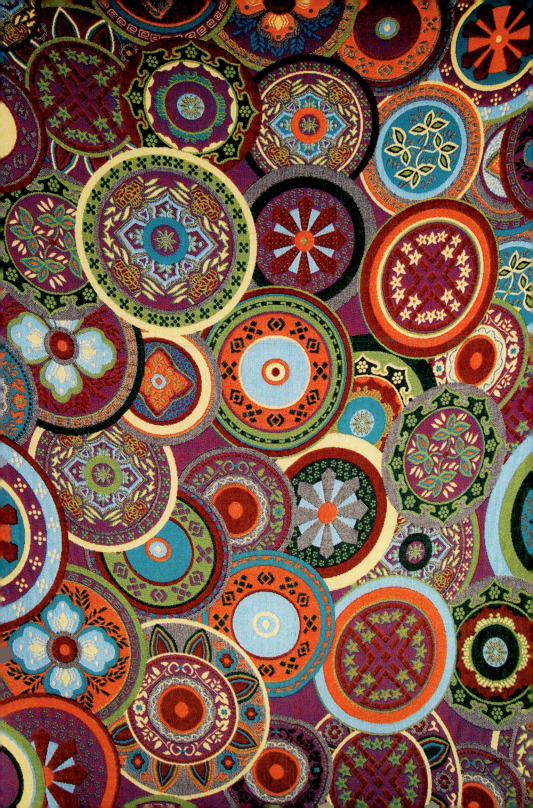

# Aloe Vera

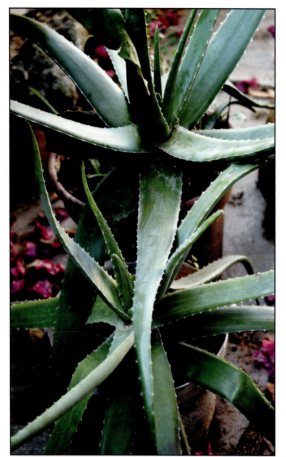

The aloe vera is native to Africa and has been prized for its medicinal and ornamental qualities for centuries. It is related to garlic and there are about 400 species of it. Aloe vera grows in the dry regions of every continent. It may reach up to 1 m, has almost no stem and a rosette of large, thick leaves that contain transparent gel. Flowers are produced on a spike and vary in color from yellow to dark ocre. It is a popular house plant.

## Spanish Name: Sábila
### Scientific Name: Aloe Vera L.

When the transparent pulp is mixed with water and taken on an empty stomach it alleviates colitis, allergies and has purifying and disinfecting properties.

Aloe vera gel is nature's best moisturizer, it rejuvenates any type of skin; use it after exposure to sun, as a base for masks, and it is a remedy for minor cuts, burns, and rashes. It is also effective against fungal infections and ringworm.

Aloe vera clear gel is by far the most efficient healing product in nature. It is a stimulant for the immune system and has strong anti-inflammatory, anti-bacterial and anti-viral properties.

Aloe vera gel applied directly on hair or scalp conditions and provides nutrients.

Fresh Aloe gel applied to the skin lightens sun and age spots and smoothens scars.

Taking fresh aloe vera juice internally cleanses the blood and allows it to deliver nutrients and oxygen to the cells more effectively.

**Not recommended for pregnant women and children.**

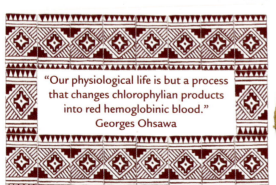

"Our physiological life is but a process that changes chlorophylian products into red hemoglobinic blood."
Georges Ohsawa

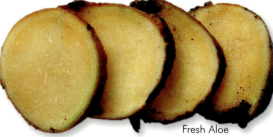

Fresh Aloe Vera root

# garden plants

Aloe juice is rich in calcium, contains 19 amino acids, enzymes, sodium, manganese, phosphorus, magnesium, potassium, vitamins C, B1, B2, and A. However, it cannot be taken in combination with any other herb, alcohol or coffee and only for the maximum of 5-7 days. After a few days of rest it may be taken again if necessary, but never for an extended period of time and **always with caution and best under supervision of experienced herbalist.**

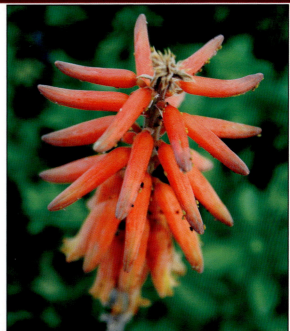

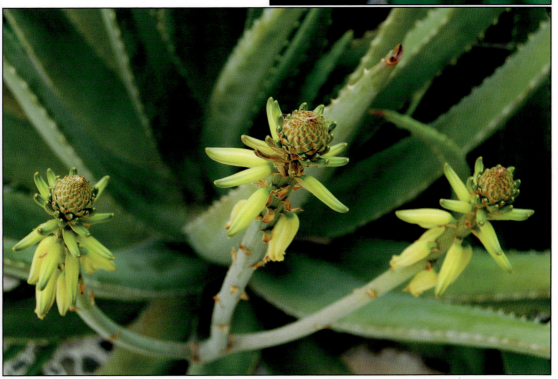

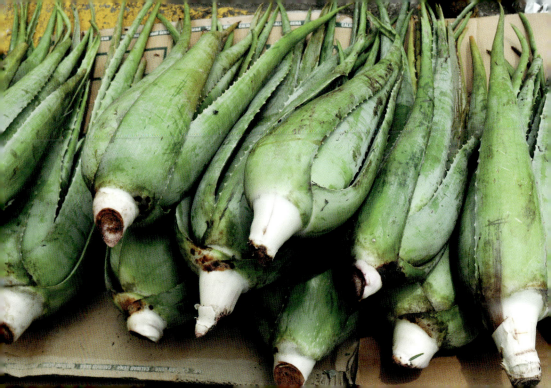

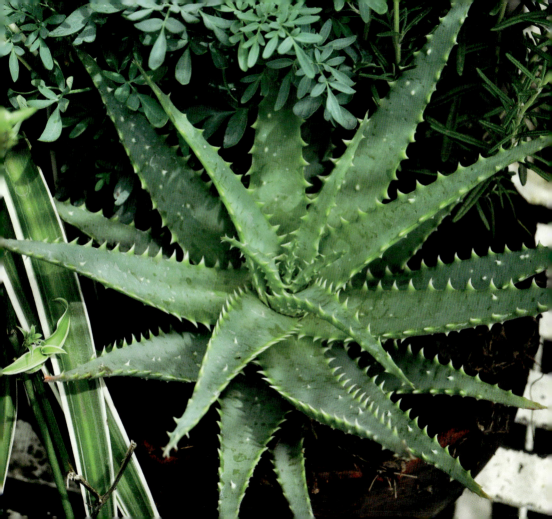

# Basil

## Spanish Name: Albahaca
### Scientific Name: Ocimum basilicum L.

Basil has a diuretic and sweat inducing effect; an infusion of leaves is good to use during fevers.

For stomach aches and intestinal parasites a handful of leaves is boiled for 2 minutes, strained, and the liquid is taken slightly warm during several days.

Local women use an infusion from the entire plant for menstrual pain, retained menstruation and to facilitate childbirth.

An infusion made with 10 leaves in 1 cup of water is an effective mouth rinse for sore gums, and a basil leaf applied over an ulcer in the mouth will bring some relief.

As a capillary tonic or to prevent hair loss, boiled leaves are made into a paste and rubbed into the scalp or added to water for a hair rinse.

For earache put one drop of juice on a cotton ball into the affected ear.

Leaves mashed in a little water can be used to dry pimples.

Leaves in poultice applied on the forehead are believed to bring relief for headaches.

Leaves dried and powdered are a remedy for inflammation resulted from embedded worms or larvae.

Basil is a delicious herb native to India, Pakistan and Thailand. It grows from 20 to 60 cm tall. There are purple and green garden varieties, with white or purple flowers. Basil likes a lot of sun and rich dry soil. The word basil comes from the Greek word βασιλευς, meaning "the king". Medicinally the whole herb, both fresh and dried, is used.

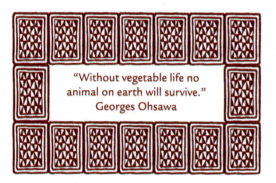

"Without vegetable life no animal on earth will survive."
Georges Ohsawa

# garden plants

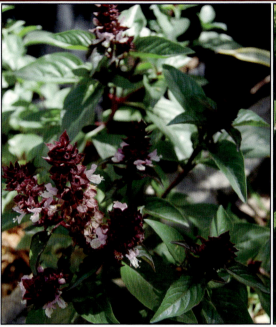
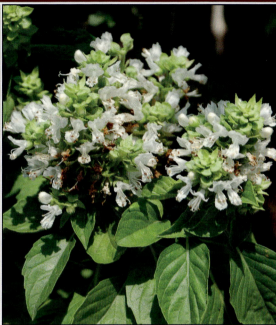

Basil essential oil has anti-bacterial, anti-inflammatory and anti-viral properties. It is a good remedy for digestive spasms and flatulence. 2-3 drops of the essential oil in a tsp. of honey is taken 3 times a day. Using basil in your food will reduce anxiety, help with insomnia, and is beneficial for muscle cramps and contractions.

Mediterranean and Indochinese cuisines frequently use basil, combining it in many delicious variations. Try it fresh in salads and sandwiches, or to add flavor to curry, soups, sauces, baked vegetables, rice, breads, hummus, pasta, pizza or omelettes.

Dried seed pod

## Salt
### Sal

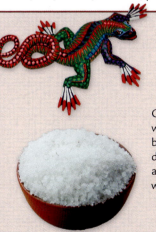

Cooking with salt produced in a traditional way not only complements taste and flavor, but adds important trace minerals to your diet. The evaporation process starts naturally and continues for several months, after which salt is hand harvested and ground.

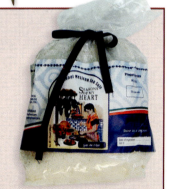

Gourmet salt from the Isthmus of Tehuanteopec used in the Seasons of My Heart cooking school in Oaxaca.

# Black Bean
## Frijol Negro
### Phaseolus vulgaris

There are many different varieties of legumes, of which black bean is one of the most widely used in Mexico. It is believed to be of American origin. The plant is not taller than 1 m and grows very easily in poor soil.

All beans are very rich in proteins and are an important ingredient in many traditional regional dishes. While dry black beans are very common, fresh beans, called *xpelón,* are a delicacy typical for the Yucatan Peninsula. They are sold at markets in bunches and the pods are about 20 cm long. Beans are delicious in soups, salads, salsas, marinades and in moderate amounts may be eaten raw right out of the pod.

Fresh beans are usually purple and green

Dried beans turn black

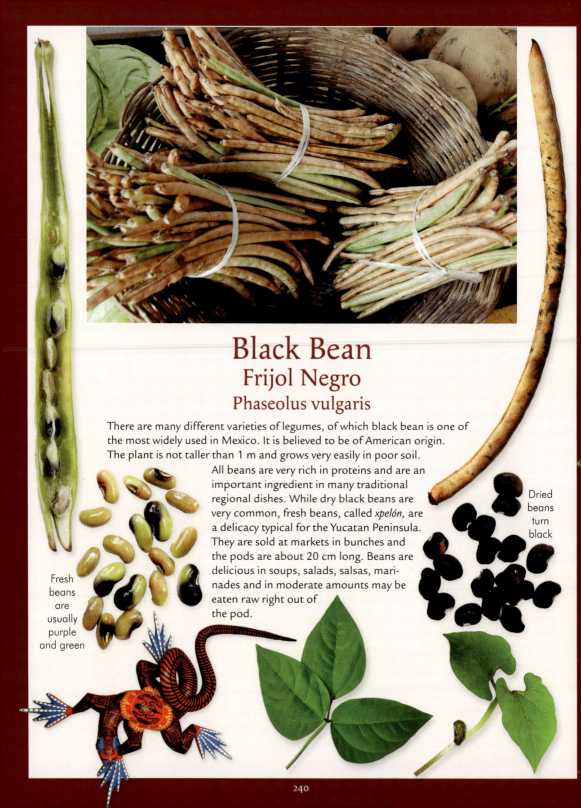

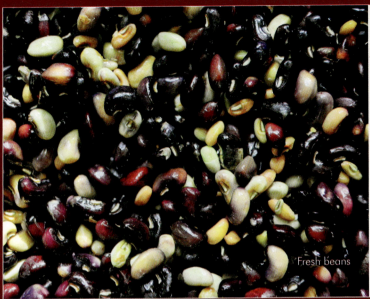
Fresh beans

## Huaraches & Empanadas

*Huaraches* are oblong *tortillas* topped with beans, nopal, mushrooms, chiles, sour cream and salsas.

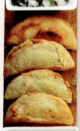

*Empanadas* are stuffed with beans or cheese

# Lima Bean
## Habas
### Vicia faba

Lima beans are the largest in the legume family and are used dry and fresh. Fresh pods are pinched with a fork and cooked in slightly salty water to be served as a side dish with butter or dressing.

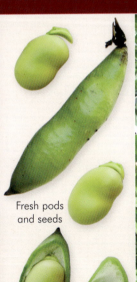
Fresh pods and seeds

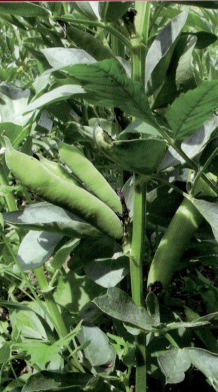

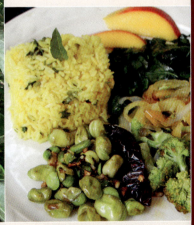

Right: Stir fried fresh lima beans with roasted garlic and *chile pasilla* marinade complement a dish of saffron rice and steamed vegetables.

# Chaya

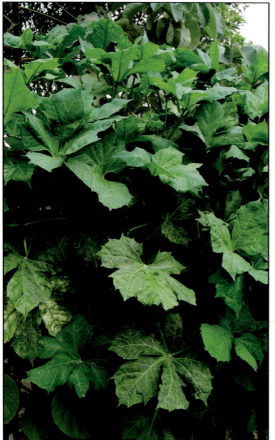

**SPANISH NAME: CHAYA**
**SCIENTIFIC NAME: CNIDOSCOLUS CHAYAMANSA**

An infusion of fresh leaves is beneficial for people with diabetes and has a diuretic effect. Corn silk and bitter cane can be added to the same infusion to expel kidney stones.

Due to its high fiber content, including chaya in your diet will promote cleansing of the intestines.

Cooked leaves may be used for rheumatism and applied on swollen joints as a poultice.

White resin from the stem may be used on pimples or to open skin cysts.

**DO NOT USE ALUMINUM CONTAINERS** to cook or store chaya. Raw chaya leaves contain a high content of hydrocyanic acid, so no more than 5 RAW leaves may be eaten per day. Only 1 minute of boiling or cooking destroys most of the acid.

Chaya, a Mayan miracle plant, is a shrub reaching a height of about 2-3 m, very common in the Yucatan. It contains very high amounts of vitamins A, B1, C, proteins, minerals, especially calcium, iron and phosphorus and is also very high in carbohydrates and fibers. Introducing chaya leaves into your diet will have beneficial effects upon digestion, circulation and the respiratory system. It is believed to improve vision, memory and brain function and combat arthritis and diabetes. It is best to use young, tender leaves that may be harvested as soon as they are around 5 cm in width. Chaya leaves are used fresh and keep well when refrigerated. Trimming encourages new growth.

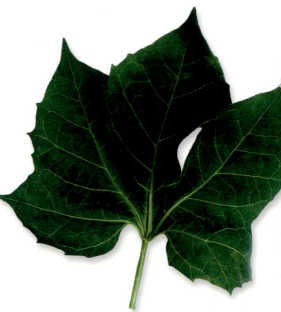

> "If you eat in good proportions you can still get sick from eating too much. Quantity changes quality."
> Georges Ohsawa

# garden plants

There are several types of chaya, most of which are edible, however wild chaya is rarely eaten because of its stinging hairs.

Chaya branches 20 cm to 1 m long may be cut off the bush and planted in the soil. They take in easily and grow roots quickly.

Leaves cut in thin layers may be added to soups, casseroles, corn dough, spaghetti sauces, salsas and salads without affecting the taste. The tender ones may be used in omelets, salads or as garnish. The larger ones are best chopped and cooked.

Fresh chaya leaves are also used in drinks. One popular local recipe includes orange juice, pineapple juice, seeded guayaba halves, a few leaves of chaya, and a little water. Blend all until smooth. Optional: ice cubes, honey.

Next page, left: Chaya leaves mixed in the traditional *nixtamal* corn dough and made into *gorditas de chaya* are another typical local favorite. Most often you find them in the markets or street corners of small Mayan towns. They are made at home and are usually stuffed or plain, served with salsa and dry and salty cheese cotija.

Next page, right: Warm chaya salad with fresh mango and roasted chives.

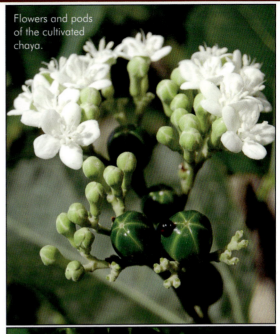

Flowers and pods of the cultivated chaya.

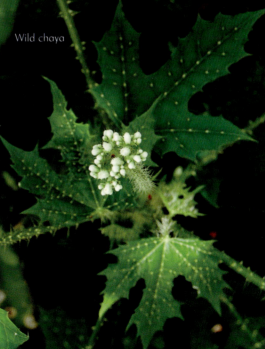

Wild chaya

Above: Spiky hair on the stem and leaves of the wild chaya make it easy to recognize.

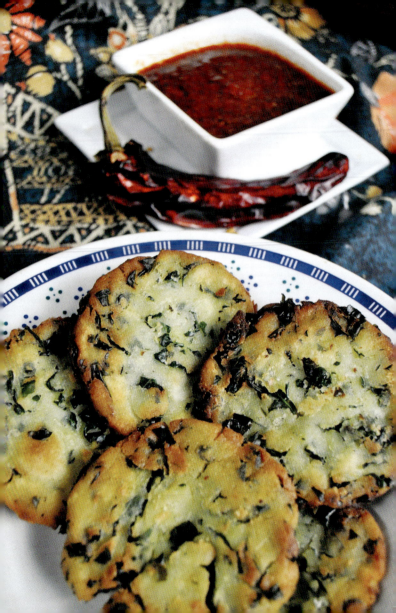

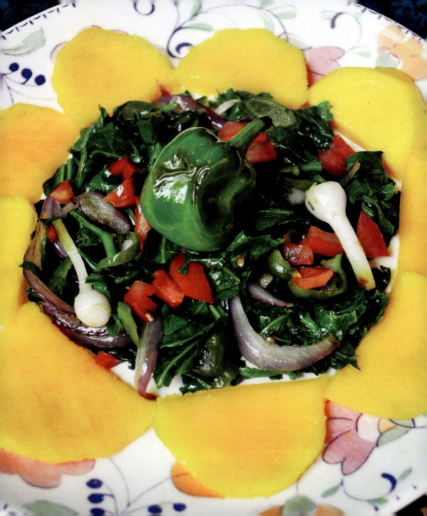

# Chiles

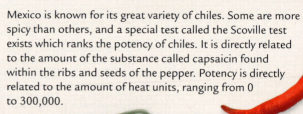

*Habañero*

*Chile de Arbol*

Mexico is known for its great variety of chiles. Some are more spicy than others, and a special test called the Scoville test exists which ranks the potency of chiles. It is directly related to the amount of the substance called capsaicin found within the ribs and seeds of the pepper. Potency is directly related to the amount of heat units, ranging from 0 to 300,000.

*Xcatic*

*Poblano*

*Serrano*

*Jalapeño*

The seeds and soft flesh that surrounds them are the most spicy part in the chile. To reduce the effect, remove it. To reduce the effect even further, soak seeded chiles in a strong solution of salty water for 10 minutes before using them.

## Chiles Rellenos

## Stuffed Peppers

This dish can be made with a wide variety of ingredients. Most commonly chiles *xcatic, poblano* or *morón* are stuffed with cheese, dipped in egg and batter and fried. Baked stuffed peppers are a healthy and delicious option.

Combine together finely chopped carrots, onions, mushrooms, cheese and cilantro. Mix and season with black pepper and salt. Fill prepared and seeded peppers of your choice and top with a teaspoon of shredded cheese. Bake for 20 minutes at 150-175C until soft. Serve warm separately or accompanied by rice, beans, tortillas and salsas.

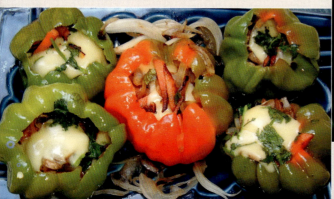

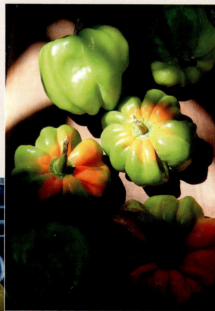

mild peppers
cheese
mushrooms

carrots
onions
cilantro

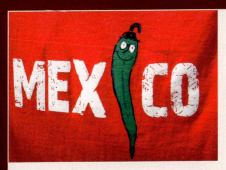

## Culinary Uses

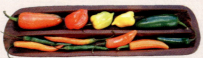

Mexico is famous for many different varieties of chiles, prepared into an amazing assortment of regional dishes and sauces, or salsas. Chiles *xcatic*, *habañero* and *morón* are the most commonly grown in small villages of the Yucatan.

## Salsa Morita

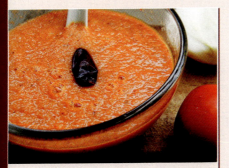

2 dry chile morita    1 onion
3 tomatoes    salt
1 tsp. extra virgin olive oil

Oil and roast whole tomatoes, halved onions and chiles. When soft, blend or mash manually in *molcajete*, adding a pinch of salt. Serve chilled or warm with tacos, enchiladas, nachos, *polkanes*, omelettes, pasta, rice an salads (above).

Below: Blue corn *panuchos* with beans, cheese, onions and salsa morita.

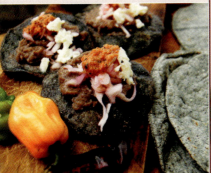

## Molcajete

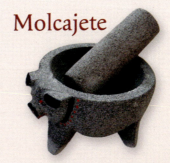

The *molcajete*, a traditional tool for grinding, is as popular today as it always was and almost every Mexican household has one. It is used to grind dry chiles and spices, to mash roasted salsa ingredients or to serve traditional dishes. *Molcajetes* differ in size, material and shape.

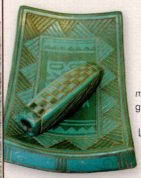

Unlike the *molcajete* which is bowl shaped, the *metate* has a flat grinding surface.

Left: Decorative *metate*.

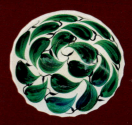
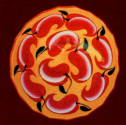
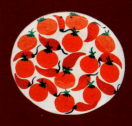
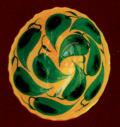
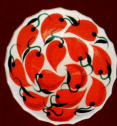
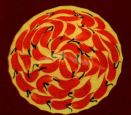

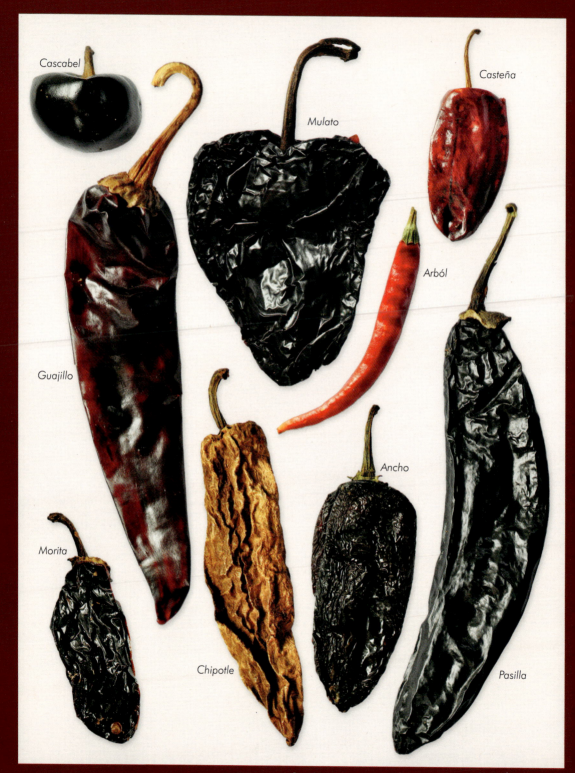

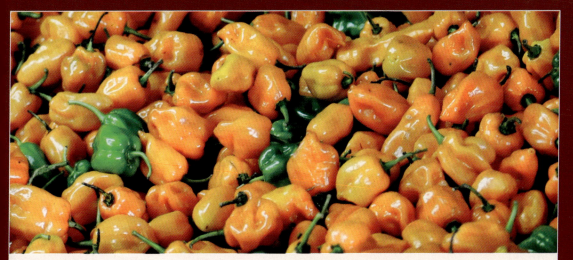

# Chile Habañero
## Capsicum chinense

The *habañero* chile originated in the Yucatan Peninsula and in the XVI century spread rapidly around the world. When ripe it can be red, orange, white, black or brown. Black *habañero*, a variety that takes much longer to mature, has a distinct flavor and is extremely spicy. The *habañero* was exported and sold at the markets in Havana, which is believed to have contributed to its name. *Habañero* chile plants like sunny spots and dry soil. When overwatered they produce very bitter fruit.

### Lime & chile salsa

Finely chopped pieces of *habañero* and cilantro are added to lime juice with a pinch of salt. It is a very liquid and spicy salsa used in very small amounts.

### Chile, avocado & tomatillo

A small amount of *habañero*, 1 avocado, 2 green tomatoes, cilantro, salt and a glass of water are blended together into a think green paste. It may be served as salsa or cold soup depending on consistency

### Chile & onion roasted salsa

Chile *habañero*, green tomato, onion, and 1 clove of garlic are roasted and blended with an addition of lime juice and a pinch of salt.

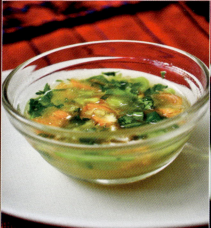
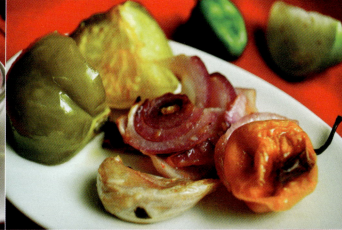

# Garlic

## Spanish Name: Ajo
### Scientific Name: Allium sativum L.

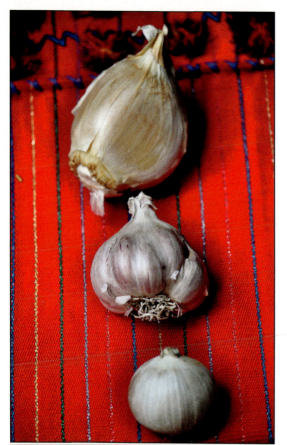

Garlic syrup is an invaluable medicine for asthma, hoarseness, coughs, and other minor respiratory disorders because it is an excellent expectorant.

An old recipe for syrup prescribes boiling garlic bulbs until they are soft, straining, and then adding some vinegar and honey and boiling it slowly to syrup consistency. Syrup is then poured over the boiled bulbs and refrigerated in a glass jar. Each morning a clove may be taken and a teaspoon of the syrup.

It may be used raw to rub on scorpion, bee or mosquito bites.

Raw garlic juice diluted with boiled water has antiseptic properties and may be used externally to clean cuts and infected areas.

Garlic is used in ointments and lotions externally due to its anti-septic and anti-bacterial properties. Crushed garlic is extremely potent and applied directly on the skin will cause burns and blistering.

For dry cough and to facilitate expectorant activity a deep penetrating carrier oil is mixed with a small quantity of crushed garlic or garlic oil and applied carefully on the chest and between the shoulder blades to provide temporary relief.

Chewing a clove of garlic and swallowing it helps with all kinds of nausea.

Garlic juice on a Q-tip may be applied on pimples and acne.

For sore throat a gargle mix is made with a little garlic juice and vinegar in warm water.

Garlic is another very ancient member of the same family as onion and it is believed to be native to Eurasia. The word garlic is Anglo-Saxon; *gar* (spear) and *lac* (plant). Garlic likes sun and thrives in rich, well irrigated soil. There are many varieties of *Allium* and some species have sweet smelling flowers.

"When human blood is permeated with herbal nutrients, the germs in the body will starve to death, and the human body will be naturally cleansed and purified. The cleansing and purifying qualities that allow herbs to last for years without rotting are the greatest benefits to be gained from herbal diet."
Dr. Stephen T. Chang,
The Tao of Sexology

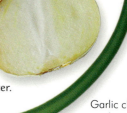

Garlic clove and sprout

# garden plants

Garlic has extraordinary medicinal properties: it is an excellent anti-viral, anti-bacterial, diuretic, expectorant, stimulant and anti-fungal. To get the benefit from garlic it is best to introduce it into the diet and use it with every opportunity.

## Baked Garlic

garlic bulbs      olive oil      salt

Peel the extra skin off the bulbs, brush with oil and sprinkle with sea salt. Bake in oven until soft. Spread on fresh bread, use in salad dressing, sauces or as a side dish to baked vegetables.

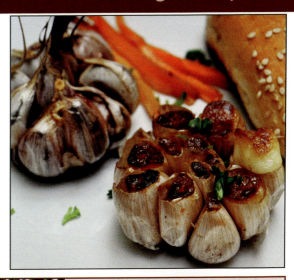

## Swiss Chard
### Acelgas
#### Beta vulgaris

Chard belongs to the same family as beets and is one of the most delicious and nutritious greens in the garden. Chard is a bi-annual plant with very long roots that reach deep underground to absorb minerals and nutrients. Chard is very resistant and does well in different climate zones. Flowers usually come out in the second year and produce seeds. Chard requires good irrigation and weeding. Chard is an excellent source of fiber, trace minerals, iron, vitamins A, B, C, and it stimulates the digestive and urinary systems. Chard is very good to steam or slightly stir-fry, or to use in stuffing for *empanadas, tamales,* pies and pizzas, raviolis, *quiches* and omelettes. Chard is delicious with other greens slightly tossed as part of warm salad or pureed with rice or pasta.

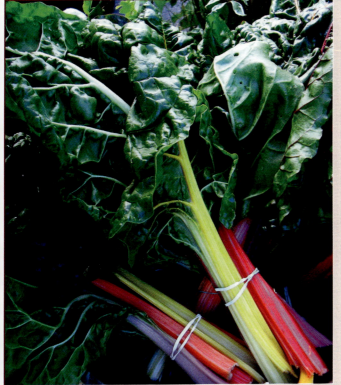

White chard is the most common in Mexico. Bright colorful varieties are well appreciated in North America.

# Lemongrass

**Spanish Names: Zacate de Limón**
**Scientific Name: Andropogon citratus L**

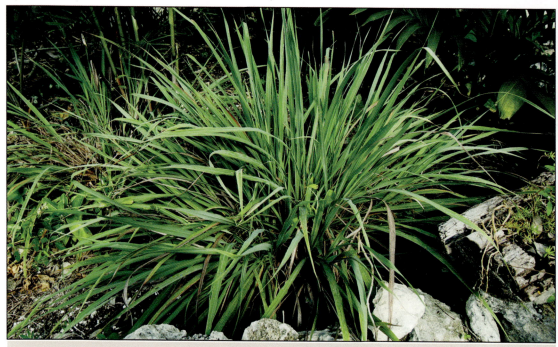

Lemongrass is a perennial plant native to tropical parts of Asia. It adapts easily and thrives in areas with much sunlight. Lemongrass is commonly used in teas, soups and curry. It is very popular in Caribbean and Thai cuisine.

In cases of high fever cleaned lemongrass root and a few leaves are boiled for 10 minutes in 3 glasses of water. When taken hot it promotes sweating and breaks down the fever.
For children only the leaves are boiled and the infusion is taken warm 6 times a day in small amounts while the child stays well covered.

Lemongrass stimulates appetite and digestion and is a mild diuretic; in infusion or tea it may be taken during the day.

Lemongrass infusion is also recommended as a cough remedy.

For backache and muscular spasms mash leaves and apply poultice directly on affected area. The same remedy may be applied for mild headaches.

For diarrhea an infusion of 10 g of leaves and stem in 100 g of water is taken after meals.

"Cellular, as well as mental, intelligence enters the body by way of the breath. As we can see, for any treatment to be successful and effective, it must raise the vibratory state of the entire body. By bringing fresh prana ito the body with proper breathing, not only is the frequency of the spiritual body raised, but also our individual cells are prompted to regenerate themselves and work together harmoniously."
The Divine Doctor, Joseph Michael Levry

# garden plants

Fresh lemongrass ready for infusion

## Ginger
### Jengibre
#### Zingiber officinale

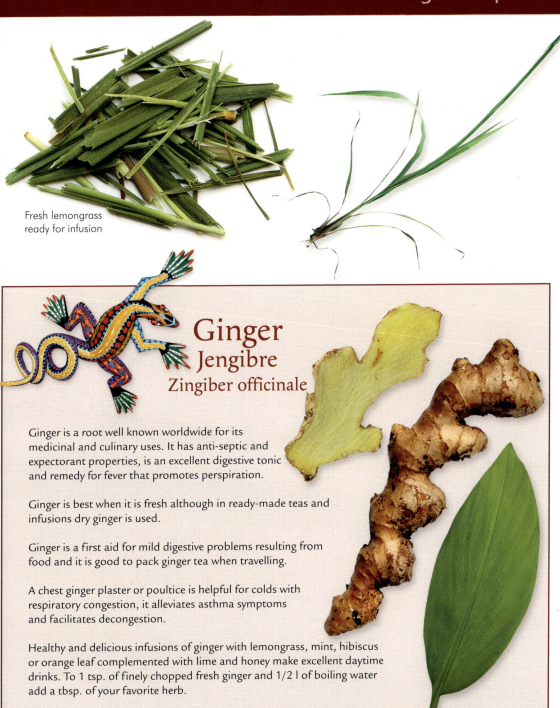

Ginger is a root well known worldwide for its medicinal and culinary uses. It has anti-septic and expectorant properties, is an excellent digestive tonic and remedy for fever that promotes perspiration.

Ginger is best when it is fresh although in ready-made teas and infusions dry ginger is used.

Ginger is a first aid for mild digestive problems resulting from food and it is good to pack ginger tea when travelling.

A chest ginger plaster or poultice is helpful for colds with respiratory congestion, it alleviates asthma symptoms and facilitates decongestion.

Healthy and delicious infusions of ginger with lemongrass, mint, hibiscus or orange leaf complemented with lime and honey make excellent daytime drinks. To 1 tsp. of finely chopped fresh ginger and 1/2 l of boiling water add a tbsp. of your favorite herb.

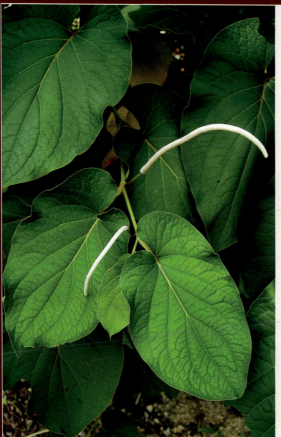

# Mexican Pepper Leaf
## Hoja Santa
### Piper auritum

*Hoja santa* is a beautiful plant that may grow a few m tall with large leaves, reaching 20-30 cm in length. It is native to Mesoamerica and likes well irrigated soil, light sun and afternoon shade. It is usually planted from the root divisions. The leaves have a very pleasant aroma and have been used both in cooking and traditional medicine. The Aztecs considered the herb a good stimulant and added it to flavor chocolate along with vanilla.

Medicinally the leaves and young stems are taken in an infusion for minor stomach problems, as a tonic for the respiratory system and to alleviate symptoms of asthma and bronchitis. Dry or fresh leaves are brewed as tea and taken during the day. Externally the leaves are used for skin infections in a poultice or as part of the ointment.

In *tamales hoja santa* may be placed over a banana leaf or corn husk wrapper to add a delicious flavor.

The flavor of the leaves makes them a very popular ingredient in Yucatecan regional cuisine. Besides flavor, the color of the leaves stays bright green when they are heated.

The leaves may be fried in hot oil and served as a garnish. When the leaves are cleaned of the hard veins they may be blended with water and added to cooking rice or a vegetable stew to give it a pleasant flavor similar to curry.

One of the most popular recipes from Veracruz is to wrap fresh fish in the leaves of the *hoja santa* and then bake it with an addition of your favorite chiles and onions. *Hoja santa* is also an important ingredient used in green *mole,* a local variation best consumed fresh made, unlike other types of *mole.* Local mole verde may contain *jalapeño* and *serrano* chiles, tomatillos, ground up green pumpkin seed, cilantro, *hoja santa,* cumin and *epazote.*

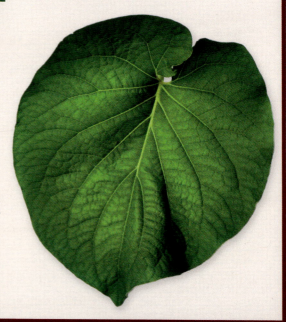

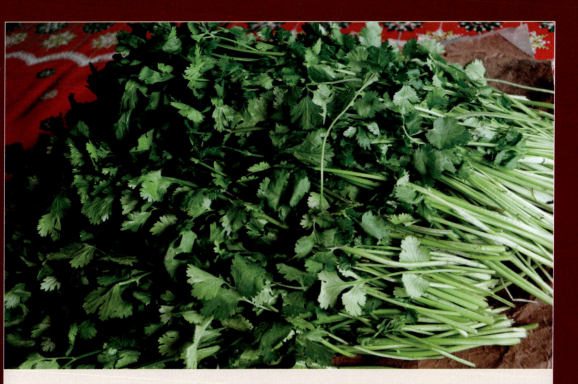

Cilantro is an annual herb believed to have originated in Southern Europe. Cilantro arrived to the American continent in the XVI century. It became one of the most used herbs in the Mexican cuisine, especially known as an ingredient in many different salsas. Like many other culinary herbs, it contains anti-oxidants that prevent the growth of bacteria in food. Cilantro pesto sauce is an excellent addition to *tamales* or *tacos*. **Cilantro may cause allergies in some people, use with caution when nursing or pregnant.**

# Cilantro
## Coriandrum sativum

Using cilantro is beneficial for the digestive system, people with diabetes, for anxiety and insomnia. The seeds have a very pleasant flavor and a diuretic effect. Tea made with 3-5 g of seeds in a glass of hot water brings relief to minor stomach aches.

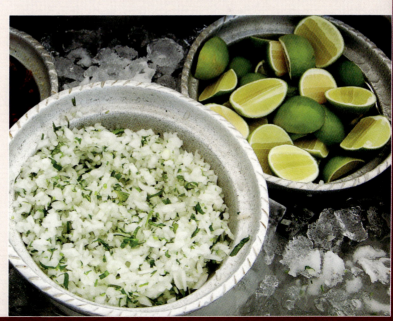

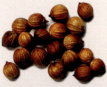

Coriander seeds

# Mexican Sage

## Spanish Name: Estafiate
### Scientific Name: Artemisia ludoviciana

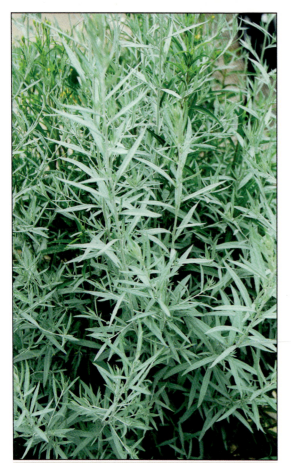

Sage is a perennial plant, about 1 m in height common to all continents. It has been used for thousands of years by native people all over the world for ceremonial and medicinal purposes. The Mexican variety has long narrow leaves and very small, brown flowers. It is very common throughout Yucatan. Both dry and fresh plant is used. Sage likes sunny spots and survives well in any soil.

Sage is used to alleviate a range of digestive ailments, as well as menstrual cramps, and is believed to be quite effective against intestinal parasites.

An infusion made with a few leaves of sage is a good intestinal tonic.

A decoction of 4 g of sage leaves in 100 g of water is made and 1 tbsp. is taken on empty stomach daily. **Not recommended for pregnant and nursing women or children.**

Sage infusion may calm liver pain when it is a symptom of gallbladder stones. A gallbladder cleanse is necessary as a follow up on this condition. Check the book Rainforest Remedies by Rosita Arvigo for instructions.

Burning sage is used as a cleansing ritual in many Native American cultures. It is believed to clear the space or personal energy field. The symptoms of the contamination commonly manifest as irritability towards loved ones, mental confusion, loss of appetite, digestive problems, feelings of discontent, loss of sleep, cold sweating and recurrent nightmares.

To prepare a tincture, dry or fresh sage may be used. Use 1/3 of herb for 2/3 parts of alcohol. Let the mixture stand for a week until the essential oils dissolve in the alcohol. The tincture may be rubbed on the skin, added to a rinse to use after a shower, or sprinkled around the house.

> "The fact is, our lives are basically ruled by unseen forces, because the invisible supports the visible. Therefore, it is in our best interest to understand the unseen forces behind the major rhythms of nature. In doing so, we can learn how to be at the right place at the right time, thus creating the best possible outcome. Success is in the timing!"
> Lifting the Veil, Joseph Michael Levry

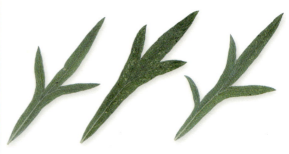

# garden plants

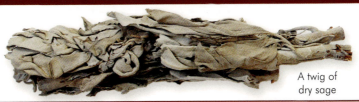

A twig of dry sage

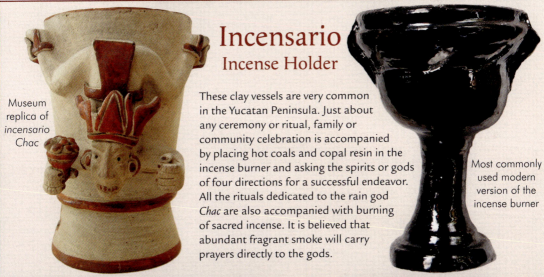

## Incensario
### Incense Holder

These clay vessels are very common in the Yucatan Peninsula. Just about any ceremony or ritual, family or community celebration is accompanied by placing hot coals and copal resin in the incense burner and asking the spirits or gods of four directions for a successful endeavor. All the rituals dedicated to the rain god *Chac* are also accompanied with burning of sacred incense. It is believed that abundant fragrant smoke will carry prayers directly to the gods.

Museum replica of *incensario* Chac

Most commonly used modern version of the incense burner

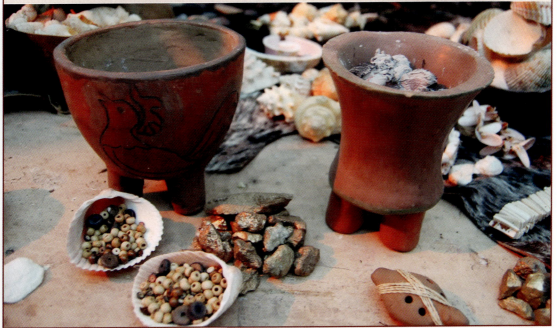

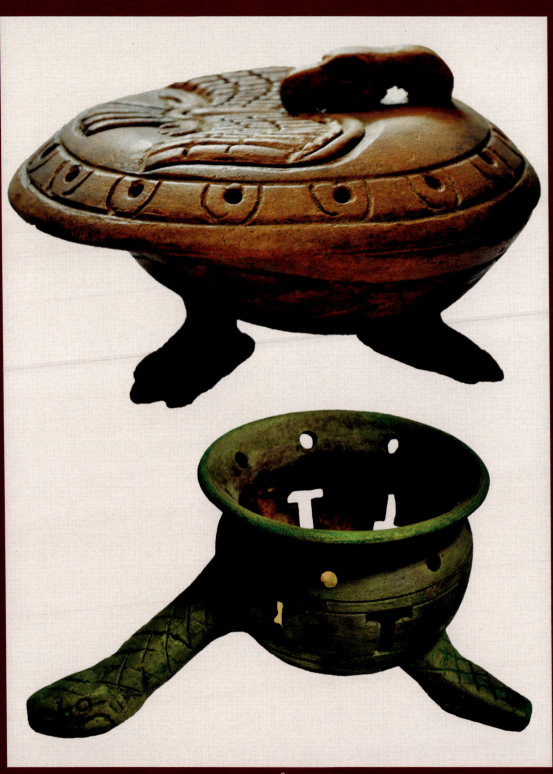

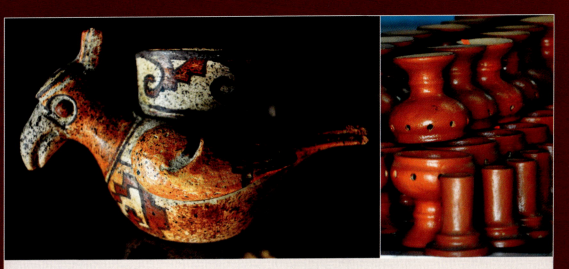

The finest incense holders were made and exported throughout the Mayan world. Simple handheld models are manufactured today for the same use as in antiquity and may be found in native markets or herbal stores.

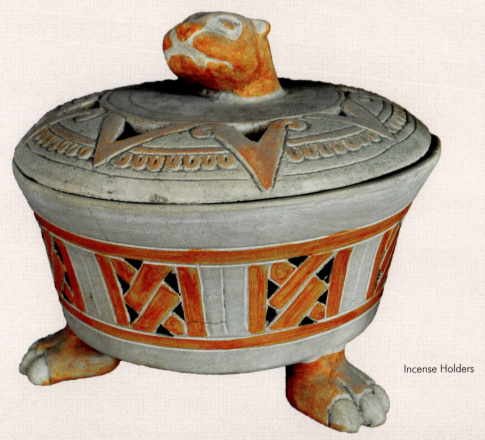

Incense Holders

# Mint

## Spanish Name: Hierba Buena
### Scientific Name: Mentha spicata

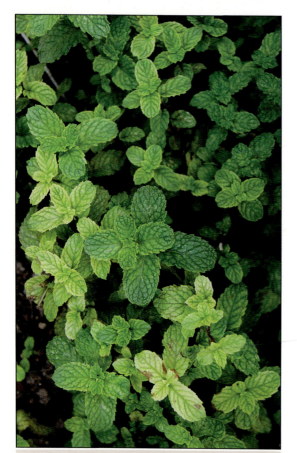

Mint is a small flowering plant. There are about 30 varieties that are very common in different parts of the world and most have similar medicinal properties. Peppermint is much more effective as a medicinal herb than spearmint, which is mostly a culinary herb. The mint family includes basil, rosemary, sage, oregano and catnip.

Since ancient times mint tea has been used as a digestive tonic, for excessive gas, stomach cramps, flatulence and nausea. It also helps in cases of mild stomach and intestinal infections.

Mint tea calms muscular spasms and is very beneficial for circulation.

Infusion with lime, honey and mint promotes nasal secretions during bronchial infections.

Very weak mint tea may be used by nursing mothers and given to babies for stomach colic and during teething.

Excessive sweating may be helped by taking the decoction of 10 g of flowering stems in 1 l of water.

To amplify its effect as a respiratory expectorant it is good to mix mint with eucalyptus and sauco and make an infusion with 5 g of each plant in dried form in a half liter of water.

Mint essential oil or juice from leaves applied directly to affected area is effective against scabies.

An ointment made with mint essential oil rubbed directly on affected area aliviates arthritis and chronic joint pain.

Essential oil applied directly on the tooth with a Q-tip may provide temporary relief for toothache.

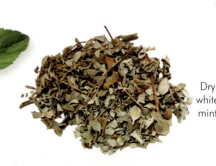

Local varieties

Dry white mint

# garden plants

### Ginger & Mint Tea

1 teaspoon of fresh or dry mint leaves

1 table spoon of peeled and finely chopped ginger

2 cups of hot water

Let steep for 10 minutes, use for colds, nausea, minor stomach infections or fever.

# Sugarcane
## Caña
### Saccharum officinarum

*Pilloncillo* cone

Sugarcane is a perennial plant that grows up to 5-7 m tall. It is native to South Asia and there are about 40 different species.

Sugarcane grows very easily and abundantly in Mexico. It is used as a snack when chewed raw or made into a drink called *guarapo*, consisting of sugarcane juice, iced water and lime.

*Piloncillo*, or jiggery, is solidified molasses obtained by evaporating sugarcane juice until it turns into sludge and then cooling it off in molds. It is a healthier option than refined sugar because it has not been stripped of its natural nutrients and processed with chemicals. It is also much less concentrated and has a pleasant taste and flavor. Try it in cooking, baking, smoothies, marmalades and sorbets.

Stalk segment

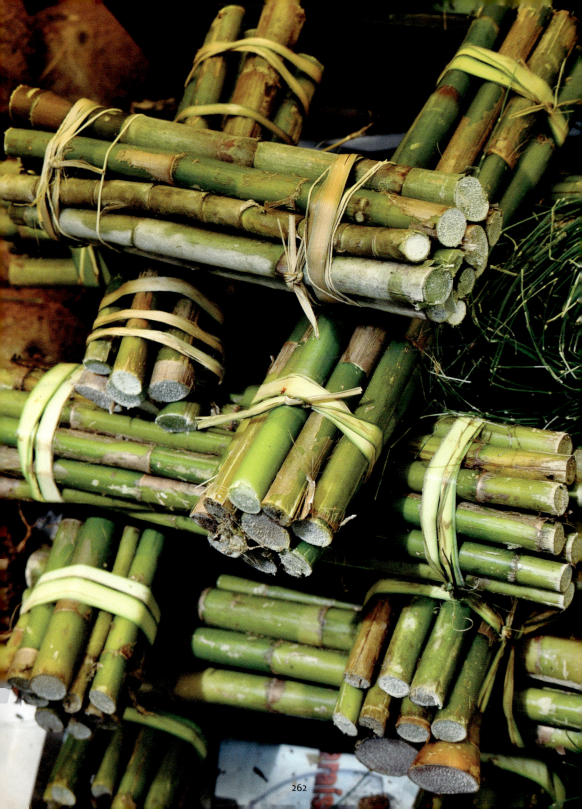

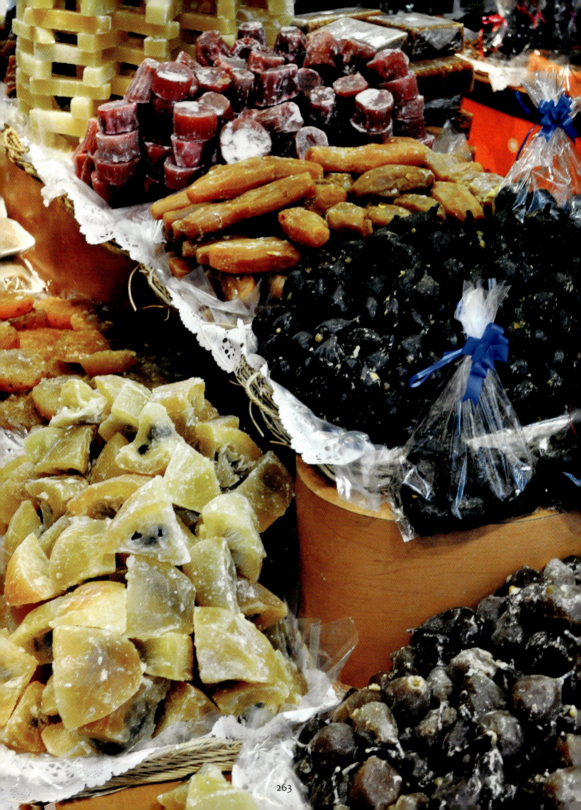

# Onion

## Spanish Name: Cebolla
Scientific Name: Allium cepa L.

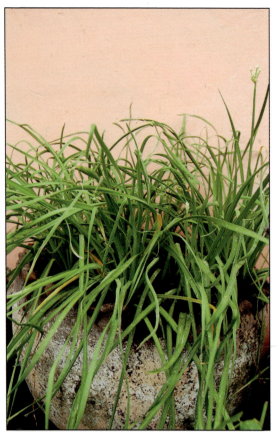

Onion belongs to the family of *Lilaceas* and is one of the oldest cultivated plants on Earth. It is believed to have originated in Central Asia and was held in high regard in Egypt, China and India. There are many varieties of onions, but they can be generally reduced to two groups with similar properties: red and white. When planting onions, leave a distance of 30-50 cm between the bulbs. After harvesting it is better to keep onions in a dry and cold place, stored in brown paper bags.

The medicinal properties of the onion have been well known throughout history. In antiquity onion was a panacea for almost every ailment, from infertility to snakebite. It was also given to athletes for endurance and strength. Rubbing onion juice on the body was believed to ward off evil spirits.

Research of the last hundred years confirmed that onion has anti-septic, anti-inflammatory, diuretic and anti-spasmodic properties. It is an excellent remedy against intestinal parasites, it stimulates blood circulation, regulates blood pressure and supports the function of the immune system. Onions contain quercetin, an antioxidant component.

Onion stimulates intestinal contractions, which improves digestion.

As a poultice onion may be applied to erupted underskin infections, inflammations, boils and warts. In many parts of the world, raw or boiled onions are used to heal blisters and boils.

> "We receive much of the energy we need from the food we eat and the air we breathe. However, the body, much like an expensive automobile, must be finely tuned if it is to run properly and utilize this energy to the maximum."
> Dr. Stephen T. Chang, The Tao of Sexology, The Book of Infinite Wisdom

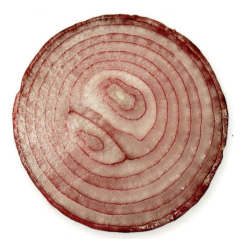

In ancient Egypt it was believed that the spherical shape and concentric rings symbolized eternal life

# garden plants

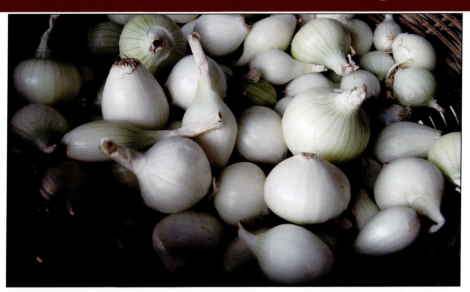

A syrup made with 250 g of honey, 1 purple onion, 7 garlic cloves and 4-5 radishes cut in cubes and left in a cold place for several days is an excellent remedy for minor respiratory conditions. Take by spoon several times a day before meals.

Against parisites in the digestive system a large onion was cut in small pieces, covered with 1/4 l of water and let to stand overnight in a cold place. Next the mix was blended and 2 tbsp. were taken on an empty stomach for 6-7 days. After a one week break, it was repeated for another 6-7 days.

In homeopathic medicine *Allium Sepia* is used for rhinnorhea and hay fever.

Raw onion juice mixed with water is a tonic for the prevention of hairloss.

Rubbing raw onion on the area affected by bee sting will bring temporary relief.

Cut a large onion in halves and rub salt in one of them, cover with another half and let stand. The juice may be applied on warts in small amounts every night until the wart is gone.

## Leeks, Scallions, Shallots
### Porros, Cambray, Chalotes

Leeks, scallions and shallots are members of the same family. The proper name of scallions is Welsh onion or *Allium Fistulosum*. Shallots are delicious when marinated in balsamic vinegar. Leeks are used cooked or baked. Creamy potato leek soup is a light and easy to make dish.

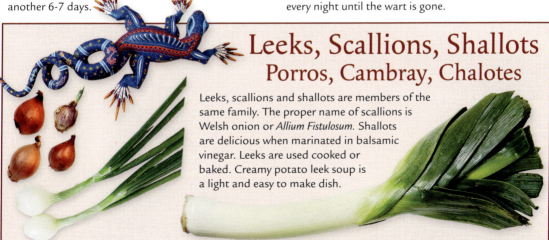

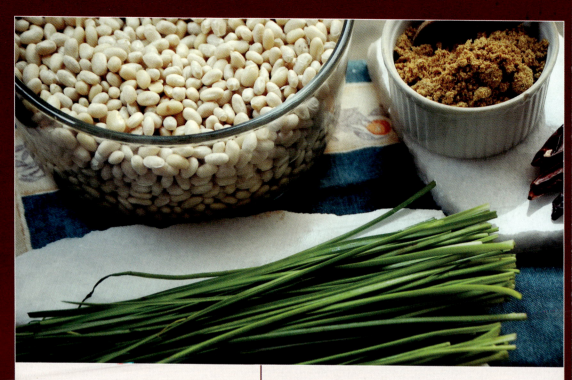

# Polkan
(*Pol*-head, *Kan*-serpent)

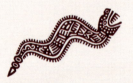

The *polkan* is a unique Mayan specialty food that cannot be found in other parts of the country. *Pol* means head and *Kan* means serpent, so it is "serpent head".

*Polkanes* are served with many different condiments that may include hot chile *habañero* salsa, raw cabbage or lettuce, marinated purple onions, red tomato salsa and avocado or green salsa.

*Polkanes* are nutritious and easy to make for lunch, dinner or to use as a picnic item that is easy to pack.

Toasted brown pumpkin seed powder

Fresh or dry chives

Cooked until very soft small white alubia beans

Nixtamal or regular corn dough

Note: White, yellow or blue corn may be used for this recipe.

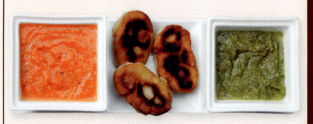

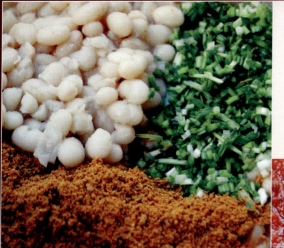

Combine cooked beans, pumpkin seed powder and cut chives and mix into a thick paste. Roll corn dough between two layers of plastic and cut round shapes of desired size. Place filling with a spoon and close up making a slightly oval shape. Fry in hot oil until golden brown. When ready to eat, slice in two halves and stuff with your favorite ingredients and dress with your choice of salsa.

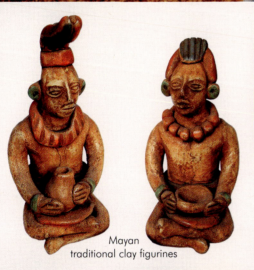

Mayan traditional clay figurines

Onions have large quantities of vitamin C and mineral salts. Pumpkin seeds are a good source of magnesium which is very important because it allows the body to utilize C, E and B-complex vitamins. It is vital for the proper function of the nerves and muscles, especially the heart.

Below left: Bite-size *polkanes;* Right: Stuffed *polkanes.*

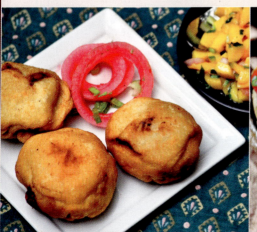
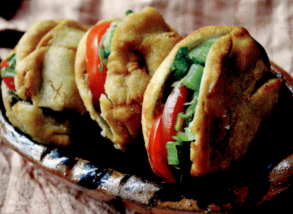

# Oregano

## Spanish Name: Oregano
### Scientific Name: Lantana involucrata

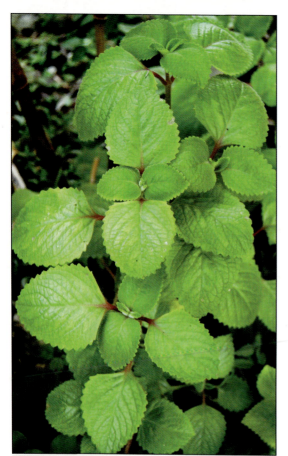

Oregano is native to the Mediterranean where it is has been an important culinary herb since antiquity. The leaves are used fresh and dry. There are many species with slight differences in fragrance which depends greatly on the conditions of the soil and climate. Marjoram is a close relative of oregano. In the Yucatan there are two most common varieties of Mexican oregano and both have a very strong and distinct flavor.

Oregano is highly prized for its anti-oxidant and anti-microbial properties.

Oregano tea or infusion is a cough remedy and is beneficial for the upper respiratory system.

Oregano used as a condiment is known to stimulate digestion.

An infusion of 20 g of dry herb for 1 l of water is a remedy against intestinal parasites and infections. It is best to use fresh plants and to take one cup before every meal for 6 consecutive days.

5 g of leaves and flowers for 1 l of water in infusion will stimulate retained menstruation.
**Not reccomended for pregnant or nursing women.**

To facilitate the cleansing of the uterus after childbirth a cup of infusion of fresh oregano leaves was taken for 7 days. The same infusion may be used to clean skin irritations and minor inflammations.

"A good appetite is essential to our life. Good appetite means happiness, good health and liberty."
Georges Ohsawa

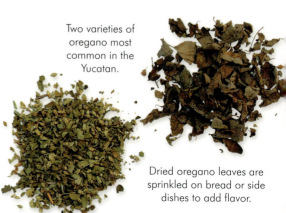

Two varieties of oregano most common in the Yucatan.

Dried oregano leaves are sprinkled on bread or side dishes to add flavor.

# garden plants

Two common Yucatan varieties of oregano are only close relatives to *Oregano Vulgaris: Lantana involucrata* belongs to the verbena family and *Plectranthus Amboinicus* (right), belongs to the mint family. It is also used more as a medicinal plant than a culinary herb.

Oregano is good to add fresh to salads or salad dressings, vegetable stir-fries and soups.

Essential oil of oregano is an excellent remedy for tropical fevers and amoebas. 2 drops of oil in a spoon of honey is taken 3 times a day.

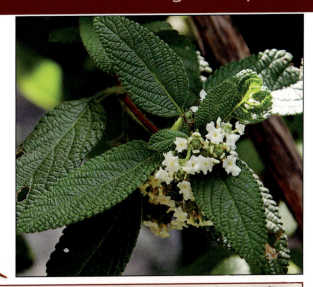

## Turmeric
### Curcuma
#### Curcuma longa

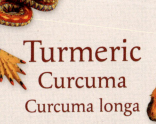

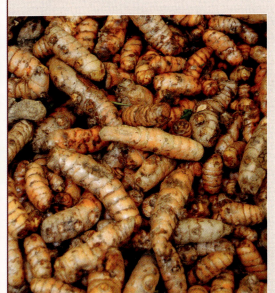

Turmeric belongs to the ginger family along with cardamon and is native to Asia. The roots are harvested, cooked for a few hours, dried and ground into a popular spice. Turmeric is part of curry spice mix and is an alternative to saffron.

Turmeric has been highly appreciated for its medicinal qualities since antiquity. It may be used as an anti-septic for cuts, minor burns and bruises as it is attributed anti-bacterial and anti-inflammatory properties. In Ayurvedic and Chinese medicine turmeric is used to treat some infections, gall bladder problems, arthritis and liver problems.

Using turmeric is believed to maintain healthy blood vessels, inhibit the growth of cataracts, help to detoxify the body, help with minor stomach problems caused by salmonella and protozoa and is beneficial for the heart.

# Jicama
## Pachyrhizus erosus

*Jicama* (from the *Nahuatl* word *xicamatl*) is a vine that reaches up to 5 m in height. The root may weigh up to 2 kg. *Jicama* is a relative of the potato family and is a popular staple food in Central and South America. It is high in vitamin C, carbohydrates and low in sodium and calories.

*Jicama* is most often eaten as a snack with salt, chili and lime, but may also be used in salads in combination with beets, cucumbers and carrots. Due to its very high fiber content jicama is an excellent cleanser of the digestive system.

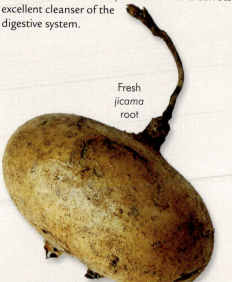

Fresh *jicama* root

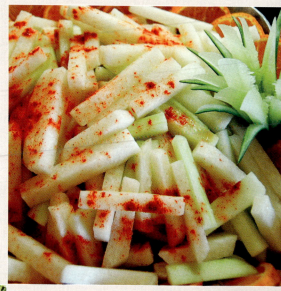

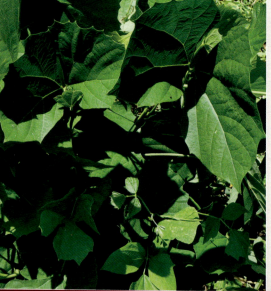

Above: *Jicama* with chile and lime.
Left: *Jicama* plant

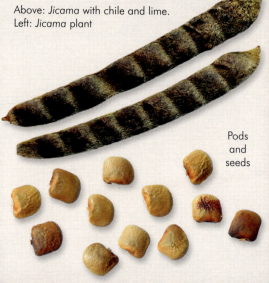

Pods and seeds

# Yuca
## Manioc
### Cassava

Yuca is a root vegetable believed to be native to South America. In Caribbean regions it was always an important ingredient in the diet. Easily substituted for potatoes in soups, stews and salsas, it may be also ground into flour for cakes, noodles and pastry. Traditionally it was ground in a stone metate to turn it into flour, tapioc.

Below: Yucca sweet rolls are sold drizzled with honey and are a popular treat easily found at the markets of small Mayan towns.

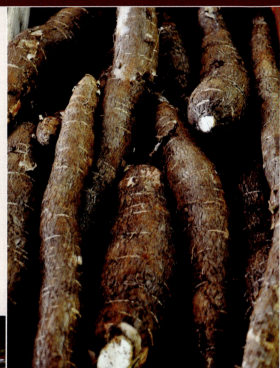

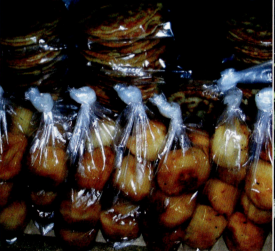

Yuca contains high amounts of vitamin C and carbohydrates. When buying yuca it is best to choose blemish free tubers. The two varieties of this tuber are the sweet, *Manihot utilissima*, and the bitter, *Manihot esculenta*, the latter being poisonous due to its hydrocyanic acid content. *Manihot esculenta* was used mainly in South America where the poison was extracted in a very complicated process.

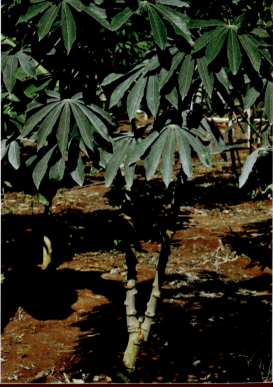

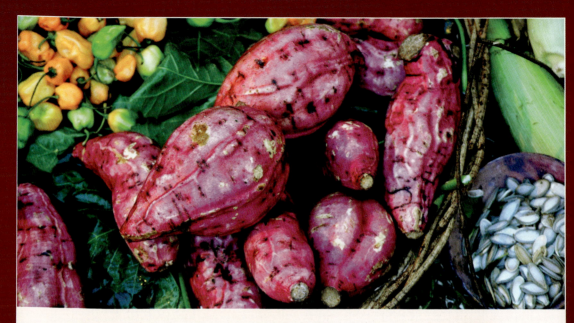

# Yam
## Camote
### Ipomoea batatas

It is not known where sweet potato was first cultivated. Archeological evidence found in Peru dates back to 2000 BC. It is a perennial plant distantly related to the potato; its tuberous roots mature in 2 to 9 months. The roots are usually boiled, fried or baked. They have a very high nutritional value and are very rich in fiber, vitamin C, A, B6, iron, calcium and protein. Young leaves may also be used in stir fries or soups. Dark orange sweet potatoes have higher vitamin A content than the ones with white flesh. In South America the juice of red sweet potato in combination with lime juice is used for fabric dyes. Firm roots without bruises are best.

Right: *Camote* puree served with blue corn tostadas & warm salad.

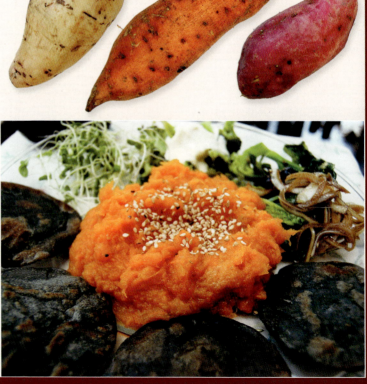

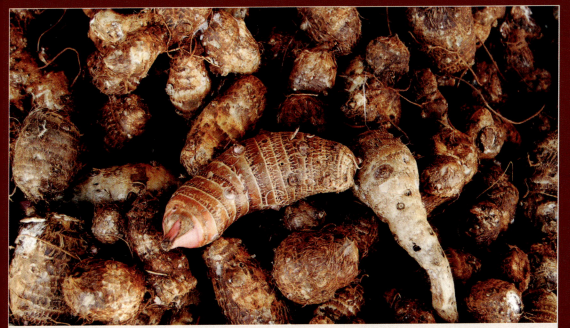

# Makal
## Xanthosoma yucatanense

*Makal* is a root of a plant common to tropical and semi-tropical climates with a growing cycle of about 10 months during which it produces an abundance of tubers the size of potatoes. The tubers are only used cooked. They have an earthy and nutty flavor and are good in soups and stews. Two other varieties of *makal* common to the Yucatan are called in Mayan *makal k'uch* and *makal boy*, with similar nutritional properties.

# Ñame

Ñame is a root vegetable used in typical Mayan Yucatecan cooking. A dish called *x-kukut makal* is a stew made with *ñame* root peeled and boiled in water until soft, then cut into small pieces. A few dried chiles are ground up together with annato seeds and stir fried with diced onions and tomatoes. All the ingredients are combined and salt and olive oil are added to taste.

This traditional dish is called Ñames voladores en caldo. Ingredients: *Ñame* or *makal* root, tomatoes, onions annato seeds, dried chiles of your choice, salt and extra virgin olive oil.

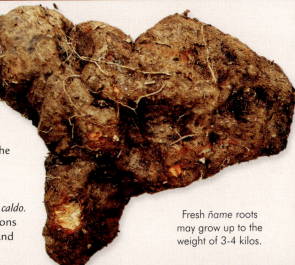

Fresh *ñame* roots may grow up to the weight of 3-4 kilos.

# Rosemary

## Spanish Name: Romero
### Scientific Name: Rosmarinus officinalis

Rosemary has a very old reputation for improving memory.

Dry leaves are burned as incense to clear the space of bad vibrations or during ceremonies and rituals.

An infusion made with fresh or dry rosemary leaves, stimulates digestion, bile production, alleviates muscular pain, is a good tonic against headaches and poor circulation. It has a beneficial effect on the nervous and reproductive systems.

For people with allergic reactions or seizures pre-caution is necessary. Rosemary essential oil is very powerful, it may cause convulsions and is toxic if ingested. **Large quantities of rosemary leaves can cause adverse reactions. Do not use if pregnant or breastfeeding.**

Rosemary is also reported to stop dandruff. Make infusion and use as a hair rinse. Mixed with infusion of nettles it revitalizes scalp and prevents baldness.

Introducing rosemary into the daily diet has an overall beneficial effect because of its natural anti-oxidant properties.

In decoction it can be used as a disinfectant, as a mouth wash or mild anti-septic.

Rosemary is a perennial herb native to the Mediterranean region. It rarely grows taller than 2 m and depending on the variety may have different colored flowers, from white to blue. This herb likes dry soil and may be harmed by overwatering.

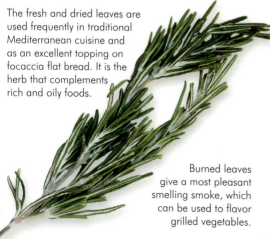

The fresh and dried leaves are used frequently in traditional Mediterranean cuisine and as an excellent topping on focaccia flat bread. It is the herb that complements rich and oily foods.

Burned leaves give a most pleasant smelling smoke, which can be used to flavor grilled vegetables.

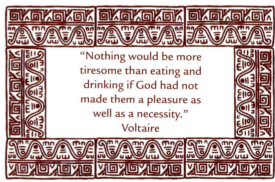

"Nothing would be more tiresome than eating and drinking if God had not made them a pleasure as well as a necessity."
Voltaire

# garden plants

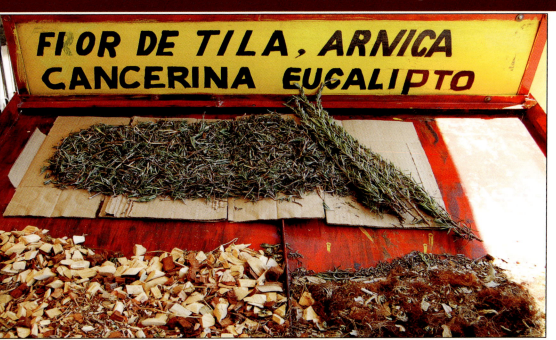

Above: Fresh rosemary put to dry at an herbal stand.

## Thyme
### Tomillo
#### Thymus ulgaris

There are more than one hundred varieties of thyme, most not more than 30 cm tall, with very small leaves and purple flowers that produce tiny seeds. Thyme is very aromatic and may be used fresh or dry for both medicinal and culinary purposes. Thyme can be grown in the garden or in clay pots. It likes dry soil and sun. Thyme has anti-septic and stimulating effects. It expels intestinal parasites, is a powerful expectorant and a good digestive tonic.

Essential oil of thyme is excellent to use for massage in cases of asthma.

Used externally thyme essential oil alleviates the effects of insect bites. It has anti-fungal properties and may be used against rheumatism and sciatica.

# Rue

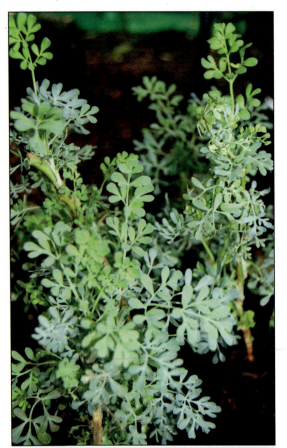

The common rue, also known as herb-of-grace, is believed to be native to southern Europe. It is very popular as an ornamental plant and highly valued for its medicinal properties and strong aroma. The rue family accounts for about 1000 species. In Mexico there are two most popular varieties that are usually planted near the house to keep evil spirits away. It is a plant of air and is traditionally used during rituals and ceremonies intended to clear the space of undesired energies.

"In the old days the sages treated disease by preventing illness before it began, just as a good government or emperor was able to take the necessary steps to avoid the war."
Huang Di, The Yellow Emperor

## Spanish Name: Ruda
### Scientific Name: Ruta graveolens L.

Rue is a bitter, aromatic stimulant that has been used since time immemorial.

Rue is used in infusion in very small quantities and under the supervision of an experienced herbalist. 3-5 g of leaves are used for 1 l of water as a remedy for retained menstruation, intestinal parasites, nervous conditions, and to prevent epileptic attacks.

Mayan midwives use rue in very small doses during childbirth to facilitate contractions.

8 g of rue boiled in 200 g of water is effective against lice as a hair rinse. Shredded avocado seed may be added to this mixture.

Rue tincture may be used as a rub for muscular pains, back pain and minor traumas.

A poultice of rue is good for sciatica, pain in the joints and gout.

Fresh rue can be used as an insect repellent if rubbed between the hands to release the essential oils.

For abssesses mashed leaves of ruda are applied directly on the area, then covered with gauze.

**Rue is a toxic herb.**

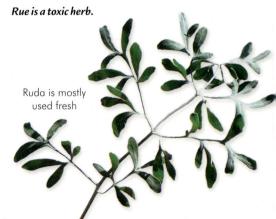

Ruda is mostly used fresh

# garden plants

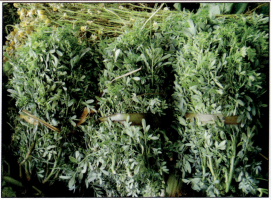

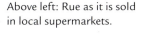

Above left: Rue as it is sold in local supermarkets.

Right: Rueflowers.

Far Right: Another variety of rue most commonly found in the small Mayan towns of Yucatan. Instead of rounded leaves, it has pointed ones.

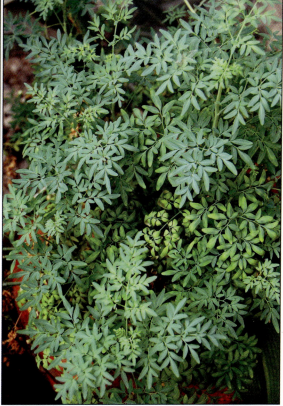

## Obsidian Tools

Obsidian tools were among the discoveries in the oldest known settlements in Guatemala dating to 10000 BC.

Obsidian is a volcanic glass, in shades from translucent grey to deep black. It is not very hard and relatively easy to carve because it is predictable where it will break. There is no Mayan archeological site without obsidian. Unlike jade, it was available to all households and was used in agriculture, food preparation, rituals, arts, jewelry, hunting and decoration. Natural deposits of obsidian are located in the Mayan highlands, from where it travelled everywhere in the Mayan world along well established trade routes.

Obsidian blades are very sharp and "cutting edge" medical technology employs this material for making scalpels used in heart surgeries.

# Tepin Chile

## Spanish Name: Chile Tepín
### Scientific Name: Capsicum annuum

Chile mash or hiltepin is native to the American continent and considered to be the original parent of most species of *Capsicum annuum*. The plant, which is a bush reaching 1 to 2 m in height, grows in every garden in Yucatan. The word tepin comes from the *nahuatl* word meaning "flea". Tepin chiles can be long or round in shape.

> "The principles of healing and medicine in general are difficult to grasp because many changes occur in illness and the healing process must adapt to that. It becomes difficult to know the root. The origin of illness can be so small and vague, in fact, so elusive, but the illness can still become substantial overtime."
> Huang Di, The Yellow Emperor

It is believed that picking up a fresh pepper and tracing a shape of the eye starting at the temple and returning back to it without touching the skin and then throwing the pepper behind the left shoulder rids one of pink eye.

All chiles are of dry and hot nature. They promote good digestion, kill parasites, stimulate circulation and help to clear out the phlegm from the body.

Plasters made with pepper and applied, with care not to burn the affected area, were traditionally used to treat sciatica and neuralgia.

Pepper in food heats up the stomach and is good in case of chills and colds.

A tiny dry chile called *piquin* is not so spicy, between 30,000 and 50,000 units and is similar in size and shape to tepin. Chile *piquin* is used in salsas, soups and is delicious pickled in vinegars or marinades due to its hearty, smoky flavor. When fresh it is slightly bigger in size than chile tepin and is shaped as a long narrow pepper.

The color is due to caratenoid content which was one of the first sources of Vitamin A in the human diet.

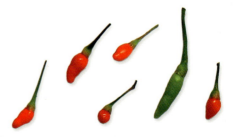

Tepin peppers are extremely spicy; 50,000 to 100,000 units. Their heat is very strong but not long lasting.

# garden plants

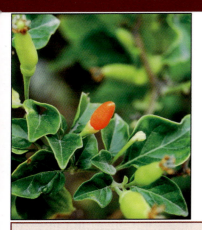

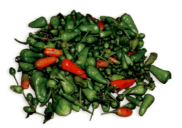

Left, center: Fresh chile tepin

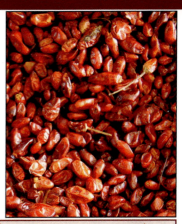

Right: Dry chile *piquin*

## Chayote
### Sechium edule

*Chayote* is a very common garden vine and a member of the squash family. It is believed to have been domesticated in Mexico and is found in markets in 3 varieties: prickly, light green and white.

*Chayote* seems to have been very popular in both the Mayan and Aztec diet. It is well appreciated all over Yucatan, in Chiapas and Tabasco and baked is a popular street snack. It is also used in stews with other vegetables, added to beans or soups. It does not have much taste or flavor so it may be enhanced with herbal oils or combined with stronger ingredients.

Tea made of *chayote* leaves is believed to dissolve kidney stones and to be a good remedy for arteriosclerosis and high blood pressure.

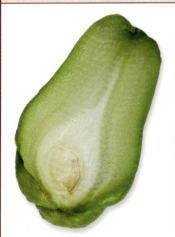

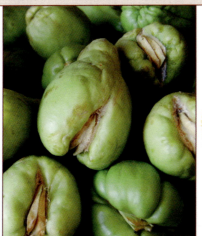

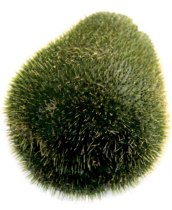

# Tomato
## Jitomate
### Solanum lycopersicum

Botanically tomato is a fruit from the nightshade family and a relative to potato and eggplant. It is believed to have been cultivated in Mexico due to its similarity to the tomatillo, or green tomato, which was a staple food in the Aztec and Mayan diet. In Europe tomato gained popularity by the XIX century. The leaves of the tomato plant contain toxic alkaloids and cannot be eaten.

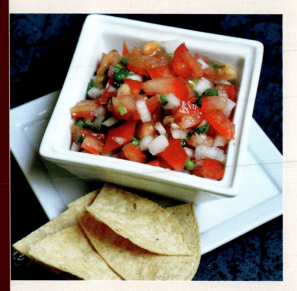

There are hundreds of varieties of tomatoes, used as a vegetable around the world in most delicious combinations. Tomatoes are an excellent source of Vitamins C, A, niacin, riboflavin, manganese, potassium, dietary fibers, copper, iron and chromium. They are rich in anti-oxidants that travel through the body neutralizing free radicals damaging to cell membranes.

Enjoying tomatoes in juice, raw or cooked, will reduce inflammation, provide beneficial effects for asthma, diabetes, protect your cardiovascular system and reduce the tendency to blood clotting and frequency of migraines. Lycopene, a caratenoid found in much higher quantities in organically grown tomatoes, has been confirmed to have anti-oxidant and cancer-preventing properties. There are hundreds of varieties of tomatoes, used as a vegetable around the world in most delicious combinations.

A popular Mexican salsa is called *pico de gallo* and includes red tomatoes, fresh chiles of your choice, onions, cilantro, lime juice and sea salt.

Many variations of warm salsas are made with tomatoes and dried chiles roasted on comal and ground up with a *molcajete*.

Cooking reduces the acidity of tomatoes and drying allows them to be preserved naturally.

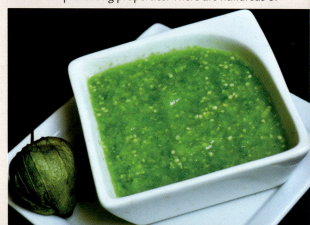

# Tomatillo
## Tomate verde
### Physalis philadelphica

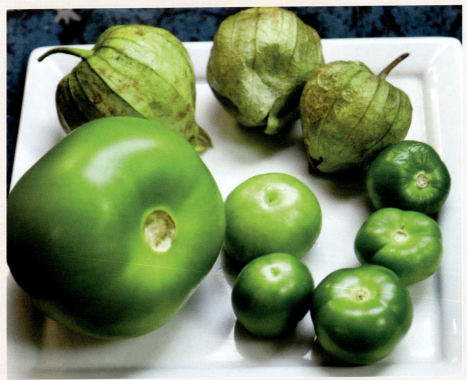

An important crop for ancient Aztecs and Maya, green tomatoes belong to the same family as the red ones. The fruit is inside a husk, which it fills up while maturing. When the fruit is ripe it remains green and the husk becomes dry and brown. The fruit may range in colors from yellow to purple depending on the variety.

Tomatillos are used cooked or raw as a main ingredient in many green salsas.

Tomatillo marmalade is also made and is delicious as a side dish to a cheese plate. When more chile is added it may be used as a relish.

A cold green gazpacho is made with green tomatillos, avocado, spicy chile to taste, cilantro, lime juice and a pinch of salt.

The fruit is high in calcium, magnesium, phosphorous, potassium and carbohydrates.

Medicinally a dry husk tea is used as a remedy for diabetes, and fresh fruit juice is used to reduce fevers.

# Wormseed

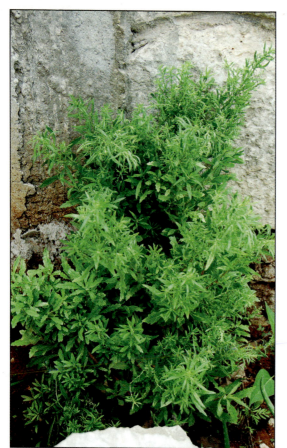

## Spanish Name: Epazote
### Scientific Name: Chenopodium ambrosioides L.

An infusion of 20 g of leaves and flowers in 1 l of water taken on an empty stomach for 2-3 days will bring on delayed menstruation and kill intestinal worms.

In combination with other herbs, *epazote* has been used for asthma and catarrhs.

Seeds and leaves of *epazote* are a good remedy against intestinal parasites.

**Caution: Not to be used by pregnant women as it has abortive qualities. In generous amounts epazote is toxic. Not recommended for small children or nursing mothers as it may cause indigestion for a baby.**

*Epazote* is a medicinal and culinary herb native to Mexico. It is a plant that is usually not more than 2 m tall and is either annual or perennial. The flowers are very small and green. *Epazote* is used fresh and it is preferable to harvest it before it starts flowering. It is very common in the Yucatan and is an ingredient in many traditional dishes.

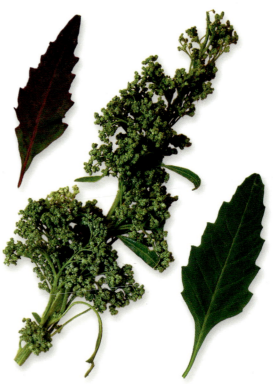

"Heaven is measured by the rule of six, and earth and humans beings are governed by the rule of nine."
Huang Di, The Yellow Emperor

# garden plants

## Culinary Uses

Most commonly epazote is used as a culinary herb for its strong and distinct flavor. Those who like the flavor use it as a leaf vegetable in tacos, *empanadas*, stews and soups.

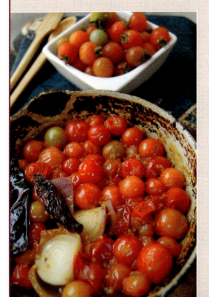

*Epazote* is good to use when cooking beans as it adds a nice flavor and has anti-flatulent properties. *Epazote* water is an ingredient in a well known Mayan dish called *papadzul*.

## Papadzul

Place 2/3 of a cup of fresh *epazote* leaves into 1 cup of boiling water and cover. Roast 3 tomatoes, 1 onion and 1 dry chile of your choice. When soft, mash or cut in small pieces. Combine *epazote* water, diced vegetables, and one cup of toasted pumpkin seed powder and mix well. Add finally chopped cilantro and serve in rolled up *tortillas* or taco style, garnished with hard-boiled eggs, purple onion and fresh chile *jalapeño*.

**Filling:**
cherry tomatoes

white onions

ground toasted pumpkin seed

dry chiles of your choice

**Garnish:**
hard-boiled eggs

purple onions

cilantro

red *jalapeño* chile

corn or flour *tortillas*

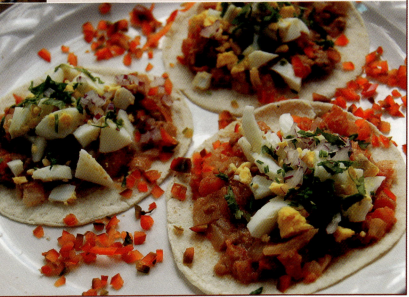

# BIBLIOGRAPHY

The Divine Doctor, Joseph Michel Levry
Lifting The Veil, Joseph Michael Levry
Alchemy of Love Relationships, Joseph Michael Levry
Rainforest Home Remedies, Dr. Rosita Arvigo & Nadine Epstein
The Cure For All Diseases, Dr. Hulda Clark, Ph.D,N.D.
The Yellow Emperor's Classic of Medicine, Neijing Suwen, translated by Dr. Maoshing Ni
The Holistic Herbal Directory, Penelope Ody
Popol Vuh, translated by Dennis Tedlock
Plantas Curativas de Mexico, Dra. Laura Samano
Plantas Que Curan y Plantas Que Matan, P.A. Carvajjal
The Tao of Sexology, The Book of Infinite Wisdom, Dr. Stephen T. Chang
Plants of the Gods, Richard Evans Shultes, Albert Hofman, Christian Ratch
The Pleasure of Eating, edited by Erin Conley
The Way of Life, Lao Tzu, a new translation of Tao Te Ching by R.B. Blakney
Humanistic Botany, Oswald Tippo and William Luis Stern
The Secret Life of Plants, Peter Tompkins and Christopher Bird
Aging, Sang Whang
The Law of Undulation, Ikuro Adachi
The Maya, Michael D. Coe
The Shaman, Piers Vitebsky
Honey, Jill Norman
Parallel Visions in Art & Physics, Leonard Shlain
Hierbas y Plantas Curativas, editorial LIBSA
El Libro Guia de la Alimentacion Natural, George Seddon, Jackie Burrow
Natural Healing, Marcia Starck
Advanced Chakra Healing, Cyndi Dale
Meeting the Remarkable People, G.I. Gurdjieff
Color, Victoria Finlay
Zen Macrobiotics, Georges Oshawa
The Book of Judgment, Georges Oshawa
Psychic Discoveries Behind the Iron Curtain, Sheila Ostrander, Lynn Schroeder
Practical Intuition, Laura Day
The Great Book of Hemp, Robinson
The Blueprints for Immortality, Harold Saxton Burr
An Archeological Guide to Mexico's Yucatan Peninsula, Joyce Kelley
Chemotyped Essential Oils And Their Synergies, Dr. A. Zhiri - D. Baudoux
Mexico Mystique The Coming Sixth world of Consciousness, Frank Waters
Bruce Lee, www.brucelee.com
Medicina Maya Tradicional, Hernán García, Antonio Sierra, Gilberto Balam

# ALPHABETICAL LIST OF RESOURCES

Arte y Decoración Maya, Ticul, Yucatan, pages 118-122, 167-168, tel. 997-972-1316,

Banyan Tree Spa Mayakoba, Playa del Carmen, Q. Roo, www.banyantreespa.com

Caracol Mexican Folk Art, pages 89-90, 104, 109, 154-155, 159-160, www.caracolmexicanfolkart.com

Delicias del Sur, Mérida, Yucatan, pages 10, 28, 30 tel. 997-975-0252

Eco-Museo del Cacao, Plantacion Tikul, www.ecomuseodelcacao.com

Hacienda Tres Rios, The Tres Rios Nature Park, pages 9-12, 37-40, 139, www.tres-rios.com

Hacienda Henequenera, Xcaret, Q. Roo, pages 150-151, www.xcaret.com.mx

Hamacamarte, pages 156-158, tel. 984-873-1338, www.hamacamarte.com

Ki'XOKOLATL, Merida, Yucatan, pages 51-52, www.ki-xocolatl.com

Librería Mundo, tel. 984-879-3004, libreriamundo@prodigy.net.mx

Maroma Amarte, www.amartemaroma.com

Meliponario, Xel-Ha, Q. Roo, pages 131-132, www.xel-ha.com.mx

Semilla de Dioses, semilladedioses@hotmail.com

Xcaret, Q. Roo, pages 42, 45-46, 140-142, 113-114, 161-162, 177-180, www.xcaret.com.mx

# INDEX

**A**
acelgas 212
achiote 125-126
agave, blue 151-152
agave, henequen 145-150
agave, Xcaret, 149-150
alebrijes 89-90
aloe vera gel, root 197-198
annato 125-126
anona tree fruit, white, red 3-4
arnica 127-128
avocado 63-64
avocado with asparagus salad 64
ayoyote 172

**B**
baked garlic 212
baked plaintain 66
banana 65-66
basil, essential oil 199-200
basket & mat making 170
bay cedar 34
bienvenida 186
black bean 201-202
black poison wood 133-134
blue agave syrup 152
boat lily 135-136
bougainvillia 137-138
breadfruit 58
breadnut 26
bromelids 139-142
bull hoof 143

**C**
cacao, criollo 15-18
caimito 19
castor oil 134
ceiba 101-104
cenote 8
century plant 145-150
Chac, the Rain God 8
chaya 203-206
chayote 238
chicle 43
chicleros 43
chico zapote fruit 44
chile habañero 210
chile piquín 237-238

chile tepin 237-238
chiles, dry 209
chiles, variety 207-208
Chocolate Museum 8
chocolate, drinking 18
chocolate, organic 18
cigars 116
cilantro 216
ciricote fruit in syrup 30
coco palm tree 21
coconut palm tree palapa roofs 24
coconut water 21
coffee 182
copal 87-88
corn 91-100
corn fungus huitlacoche 96
corn in art 95
corn tortillas, white & blue 93
corn varieties 99
cotton 153
currants 36
custard apple, infusion with 34

**D**
datura 192
dragonfruit 69-70

**E**
Eco-Museum of Chocolate 18
elephant ear 25-26
empanadas 202

**F**
fig tree 27
firebush 163-164
flamboyant 169-170
four cardinal directions 8
fresh coconut 23

**G**
garlic 211-212
ginger 214
golondrina 138
gorditas de chaya 205
gourds, decorative use 109-110
green tomato 240
ground pumpkin seed 106-107

guaje 126
guanabana 53-54
guanabana with camote 54
guayava marmelade 32
gumbolimbo tree 171

**H**
Hacienda Henequenera, Xcaret 149-150
hammocks 156-158
henequen hammocks 150
hibiscus 173-174
hoja santa 215
huano palm tree roof top 49–52
huaraches 202
huaya fruit 33
huipil 155,160

**I**
incense holders 218-220
Ixchel 121-122

**J**
jicama 229

**K**
kapok 101-104
ki'XOCOLATL 17

**L**
lemongrass 213-214
lima bean 202
lime, essential oil 72
lime, juice 71
lime, varieties 71-72

**M**
makal 232
mamey, fresh, ice cream 35-36
mango 73-76
mango fruit, varieties 73-74
mango leaves 73
mango salsa 75-76
mangrove, red 37–40
mangroves, Hacienda Tres Rios 9-12
marakuya 183-184
Mayan Ball Game 45
Mayan Ball Game court 46

# INDEX

mayan bee 129-132
Mayan ceremonial drums 113-114
Mayan ceremonial incense
Mayan clay 165-168
Mayan pottery
melipona 129-132
metate 100
Mexican pepper leaf 215
Mexican plum 20
milpa 98
mint 221-222
miracle leaf 136
molcajete 208
molinillo 18
musical instruments 111-114

### N
ñame 232
native hardwood 41
natural clay 164
Nature Park, Hacienda Tres Rios 9-12
nixtamal 94
nopal 77-78

### O
obsidian tools 236
onion, varieties 223-224
orange, bitter essencial oil, peel 13-14
orchid 175-180
oregano, Mexican 227-228

### P
panuchos 208
papadzul 242
papaya leaves 81
papaya macho 82
papaya plant 81-82
papaya seeds 81
papaya, regional sweets 80
passion flower 184
passion fruit, wild 183
periwinkle 185-186
pib 68
piloncillo 222
pineapple 140
pitahaya 68-70
plaintain 65

plaintain, baked 66
plant textile dyes 159, 161-162
pogodo tree 144
pok-ta-pok, the Mayan Ball Game 45
polkan 225-226
pomegranate, dried skin 83
pomegranate, juice 83-84
ponche 174
prickly pear 77-79

### R
railroad vine 188
rosemary 233
rue 235

### S
sacred calendar 117-118
sacred tree, ceiba 101-104
sage, mexican 217
salsa morita 208
salt 200
sanango 144
sapodilla tree 43
saw palmetto 47-48
scorpion's tail 128
sea grapes 187-188
serret liquor 28
soursop 53-54
soursop with camote 54
spanish needle 189
squash 105
squash soup with corn 108
squash, culinary use 106-108
stingless bee 129-132
stuffed peppers 207
sugar cane 222
sweet potato, camote 231
swiss chard 212

### T
tabaco 115-116
tamales 67-68
tamales, al vapor 68
tamarind 55-56
tamarind flowers 55-56
tamarind in food use 56
tequila 151-152

textiles, indigenous 154-155
thornapple 191
thyme 234
Ticul 8, 165-168, 219-220
toloache 191-192
tomate 239
tomatillo 240
tortilla baskets 96
tree of life 104
trigona 129
tropical almond 57
trumpet tree 59-60
tuna fruit 77-79
turmeric 227-228

### V
vanilla 181-182
verbena, mexican 119-120

### W
warm chaya salad 206
water lily 193-194
weaver 123
weaving 122
weaving & embroidery 155, 122-123
wild balsam apple 190
wild chaya 204
wood carving 42
wormseed 241

### X
Xcaret, Mayan Ball Game 46

### Y
yam 231
yuca, manioc, cassava 230
Yum Kaax, the God of Maiz 97

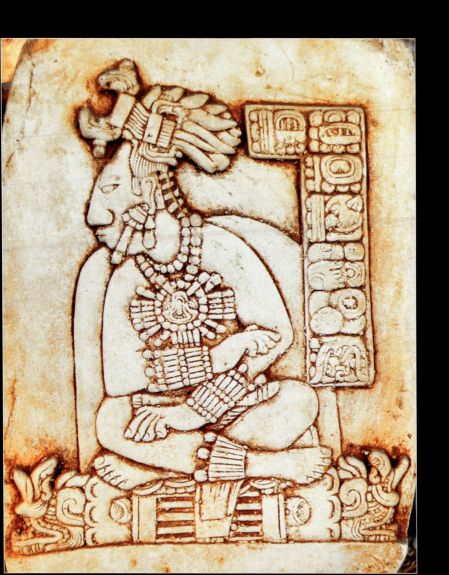

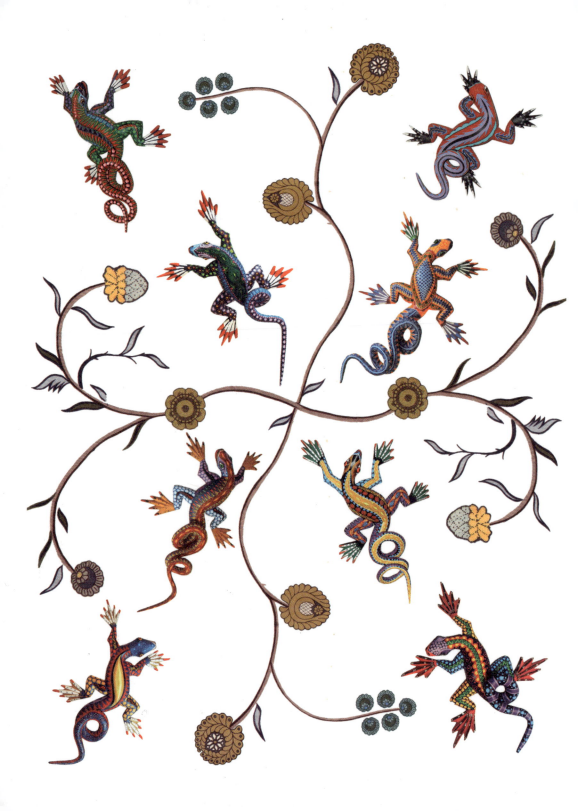